AMERICAN HEALTH CARE

A SYSTEM IN CRISIS

RICHARD COOK, Psy.D.

ISBN 978-1-63814-324-6 (Paperback)
ISBN 978-1-63814-325-3 (Hardcover)
ISBN 978-1-63814-326-0 (Digital)

Covenant Books, Inc.
11661 Hwy 707
Murrells Inlet, SC 29576
www.covenantbooks.com

To my daughters Ashley, Kelsey, and Alexa. My unwavering love for them has led to the completion of this book and my ongoing perseverance in trying to make this world a better place for them to inherit. I am forever grateful for them.

CONTENTS

INTRODUCTION

For at least two decades, the American public health-care providers, insurance companies, and good old Uncle Sam have been complaining that the American health-care system is a system in crisis and, at best, has been on indefinite life support. Indefinite life support of the system has occurred through superficial changes and intervention within health care. There might be a new piece of legislation, new health-care plans reframing old ideas, new benefits promising to bring a new direction to health care, and the like. Plenty of finger-pointing occurs with insurance companies pointing to health-care providers, consumers blaming insurance companies, and providers having unrealistic expectations from consumers and insurance companies.

In spite of these "changes," Americans complain of ever-skyrocketing premiums, difficulty with access to care, unreasonable hoops to jump through as imposed by insurance companies, declining expertise, and mounting medical "mistakes." Providers complain of escalating bureaucracy, unmanageable malpractice costs, requirements to treat the insurance company and not the patient, endless frivolous paperwork, and ever-declining reimbursement. The insurance industry complains of shrinking profits, overutilization, inability to "manage care," and unfair competition. Finally, federal, state, and local governments attempt to play the role of an insurance company while creating a bureaucracy so cumbersome that it is as complex and convoluted as the United States tax code. In doing so this bureaucracy has turned on itself. In creating its own disease process, the system has no idea of how to cure the problem let alone treat an individual symptom of the problem.

The writing of this book has come about through my twenty-nine years of involvement in the health-care system. I have been a provider, patient, consultant to the insurance industry, and taxpayer. I have been able to obtain prospective from almost every angle and perspective imaginable. More importantly, I am an American with children. I see our country torn apart by an inability to care for each other, shifting the problem to future generations, not only with regard to health care but with respect to our economic, moral, and human survival as a culture and country.

This book is intended for everyone because as the saying has long been said, there is no escaping death and taxes [and health care]. Sooner or later we all will access health care. Some of us will be fortunate enough to access it less, but eventually, we all will have to use it some extent. We are all in this boat together. It is hoped that the writing of this book will lend itself to some serious and thought-provoking considerations for identifying many of the major problems in a very flawed system. However, just identifying a problem would be in large part only to act as one more complainant in among the American fabric. It is hoped that possible solutions will also be contemplated and discussed. As a health-care provider and scientist, it has been long said that effective treatment only comes after accurate diagnosis. Hence, to address the ills of the American health-care system, there has to be an accurate diagnosis and treatment. When treating only a symptom, you never cure the illness and only avoid the inevitable, chronic illness or death.

Before I get too far, I think it is important to let you know where I sit before we talk about where I stand. I believe this is a rudimentary caveat to essentially any problem-solving situation. We identify problems and solutions from where we sit. We attempt to solve them from where we stand. I am socially and fiscally conservative. I was trained as a clinical neuropsychologist and have devoted a major portion of my adult life to assisting those in need of significant health care. Many might say that being conservative and being a psychologist is an oxymoron. In almost all instances, I would agree that is how psychologists are viewed. Most are seen as socially and fiscally liberal and anything outside of that would be sacrilegious.

In the ensuing chapters, there will be a discussion of many of the major problems of the American health care system, the pathology that drives these symptoms, and then a discussion of a new treatment course. That treatment course will be one aimed at curing the disease and not treating a symptom. A treatment course cannot be undertaken by continuing to point fingers at the insurance industry, providers, consumers, or other outside sources. A solution can only be accomplished through simultaneous intervention with each of these factions. Anything less will result in ongoing failure and the placement of a Band-Aid on a cancer.

I realize in writing this book many from each of these factions will disagree with the approach or recommended interventions. The proposed solutions may be flawed to some degree; however, a significant 180-degree course change is required. Without such a change, not only will health care continue to deteriorate but the social, political, and economic fabric of America will soon follow. I hope that this book does create some level of criticism, controversy, and dissension. If that occurs, I feel I have accomplished my goals. The objective is to shake things up. There will be naysayers, people who say it is too simple or can't be done. Remember to ask where do they sit before they say where they stand. Societally, we must abandon our apathy and push forward. My attempt to do this is through my experience, knowledge, and ideas outlined in this work. Now you must stop talking and start working for a change.

CHAPTER 1

The Insurance Industry Machine

Today's insurance industry is populated with hundreds of insurance companies offering almost countless numbers of insurance plans. There are traditional indemnity plans, capitated plans, Preferred Provider Plans (PPOs), Health Maintenance Organizations (HMOs), the Veterans Administration, workers' compensation, reimbursement through personal injury litigation, Medicare, Medicaid, indigent programs, and of course, self-pay. Each plan within each insurance carrier or payer source has a specific set of benefits or lack thereof. There is the old "eighty-twenty," the "sixty-forty," and the "ninety-ten." Then there is the Health Maintenance Organization that professes to provide "preventative care."

Preferred Provider Organizations (PPOs) are key as these groups do not provide a group of providers based on expertise or training, but rather based upon an individual provider's willingness to "accept" a particular fee schedule from a particular carrier. Differing plans have differing coverage. Plan A may cover a mammogram, while Plan B only covers 50 percent, and Plan C doesn't cover it at all. Other plans may be quite heavy into covering preventative procedures such as the mammogram, pap smear, history, and physical, while others only focus on catastrophic occurrences. Others still have no deductible, low deductibles, high deductibles, no co-pay, low co-pays, or high co-pays. Each plan has its own set of variables, placed upon the health-care equation, providing ample data for the actuarial statistician ("the bean counter") to try to account for and manipulate to the greatest advantage of the insurance company.

When these variables cannot be controlled by the insurance industry to the extent thought possible, it results in the cost side of the equation becoming unpredictable and unstable. Having countless number of plans, with endless circumstances, with countless individual patients, prediction of outcome is very difficult. In spite of these variables, insurance companies always try to be one step ahead via statistical analysis. The myriad of variables and the examination of the analysis of such is what a statistician would call an analysis of variance. Attempts are made to predict outcomes with data that cannot always be accomplished. When this occurs, it is like trying to hit a moving target while blindfolded. This occurs quite often when the insurance industry attempts to control the outcome via manipulation of the sample.

In this case, the sample is the insured group. Some carriers try to deny coverage outright by "cherry-picking" their insured. Others select only limited benefits; others limit the provider group or access to a provider via the need for a referral to a "specialist." There are a multitude of dead ends, trapdoors, and "case management" tricks the industry attempts to use. In fact, it has even become known as "managed care." Having been a provider for almost thirty years, it is clearly and always "managed cost" not care. With each attempt to control variables in the equation, there is often the introduction of artifact. Artifact is the garbage not originally intended to be part of the sample (insured group). This might be control of the providers, skewing of an insured group via "cherry-picking," and so on. One must keep in mind that the primary function of the insurance carrier statistician is to try to identify variables they believe can be measured, predicted, and controlled. Unfortunately, the human variable is usually not easily measured, predicted, and certainly not controlled. Hence, we have the hocus-pocus effect. The insurance company tries and tries but the end result in many respects is left to hocus-pocus.

With the development of various health-care plans comes added cost. There are traditional indemnity plans. These were the plans originally conceived of by Blue Cross and Blue Shield. Some people used to call them the "eighty-twenty" plan. The concept of these plans was that certain medical procedures/costs were covered in the plan. With that the insurance company paid 80 percent of the cost and the patient paid 20 percent. There was no magic to the 80 percent/20 percent formula. In fact, a plan could be sixty-forty, ninety-ten, or any derivative thereof. The plan, however, was based on a shared cost between insured and insurer.

Then there was the advent of the capitated plan. In these plans, the insurer strikes a deal with the provider to prepay the cost of health care per insured individual. The concept is to make the provider accountable for cost as the provider now takes the risk, not the insurer. If utilization is too high, the provider inevitably loses. Therefore, decisions are often made on a financial basis and not on the clinical best interest of the patient.

PPOs or Preferred Provider Organizations were yet another twist on the insurance risks formula. The insurance industry decided to enroll "preferred providers" that included physicians, hospitals, and the like. The preferred providers were those providers that agree to take a predetermined level of reimbursement for a certain procedure or illness. Nonpreferred providers were either out and excluded from the network or their level of reimbursement was even less than that of the preferred providers. Oftentimes the decision by insurance to include or exclude a provider is largely based upon if the provider is "willing to play ball."

Another insurance angle was the development of the Health Maintenance Organization or HMO. Kaiser Permanente made this model famous. In this model, the philosophy was *supposed* to be the prevention of illness and preventative care. It was believed that if this occurred, cost would be lower and health care cheaper. It hasn't occurred that way at all. Typically, within an HMO the payment is prepaid to a large extent. The insurance company has a set premium it has with each insured. Care in the plan is then provided vis-à-vis a provider/system that "employs" the provider, owns the hospital, etc. Given that the goal of the insurance company is to make money and not assure the best care, it often becomes "the fox guarding the henhouse." The insurer wants to contain costs and frequently provides incentives to "employees" to reduce cost. Insurance companies of this sort have been caught paying a bonus to physicians for ordering less test, lab work, and the like. The priority is cost, not care. Insurance companies are incentivized to provide only care that helps them reduce cost.

The Veterans Administration is somewhat a different animal. It has been a health-care system set up specifically for our armed service personnel. The hospitals, physicians, and health-care providers are employees of the government. Services and facilities are mostly paid for through the government. Occasionally, armed service personnel are allowed to obtain service outside the Veterans Administration and in the private sector. Most often this occurs when a service is not available within the system itself. Unfortunately, care is most often dependent upon huge and overbearing bureaucracy, long waiting list, and scarcity of providers and resources. The system is underfunded and has limited checks and balances.

Workers' compensation is yet another parallel system, comprised of injured employees who develop diseases or injuries as a result of on-the-job medical disease and injuries. This system is further complicated by attorneys that can directly or indirectly promote "illness" or iatrogenic-related injuries compounded by litigation. Providers are also prone to being pitted against one another by having one expert via the injured party go against the expert of the opposing employer party. It is an inefficient system fraught with adversarial opponents, secondary gain, and bureaucracy.

The personal injury system is riddled with many of the same issues as the workers' compensation system. While the injured party is not injured secondary to a work-related cause, but rather due to some third-party cause (e.g., automobile accident, "slip and fall"). Once again, it is frequently adversarial, filled with secondary gain and bureaucratic red tape.

The Medicare system, established by the federal government, for individuals age sixty-five and older and the disabled. It is generally a "fee-for-service" model but reimbursement is provided via the federal government. In large part all those sixty-five and older must have Medicare and everything that comes with such a system. Like almost all government programs, it has mountains of bureaucracy, overutilization in some areas and underutilization in others, fraud, and abuse. The program continues to have an expanse in services, yet there is no way to pay for that expansion. The expanse is most often the result of politicians wanting to appease constituents and secure their votes.

The Medicaid system and various indigent programs are state-run programs, subsidized by the federal government for individuals and children who cannot afford health insurance due to low income, poverty, or other circumstances. This program is plagued with many of the same problems as the Medicare program. Furthermore, the reimbursement to physicians, providers, and hospitals is so poor that there is an ever-decreasing percentage of providers willing to accept the level of reimbursement offered by Medicaid and associated programs. Most often the reimbursement cannot even cover their cost.

In recent years both the Medicare and Medicaid programs have collaborated with insurance companies to "assign" benefits to these programs. To some extent the government gets the monkey off of their back by allowing people to assign their benefits to a private insurance company. These insurance companies then promise to "manage" their benefits. Through marketing efforts, they will often promise expanded services not usually covered by Medicare or Medicaid. This might be dental services, optometry, audiology, gym memberships, and transportation. One must ask how such companies can provide such expended services when the government directly can't afford such benefits. Is it possible due to a population frequently on a fixed income wanting the most service possible or individuals from a lower socioeconomic and educational stratum? More about this later.

In addition to these core plan types, there are countless combinations and derivatives of them. Needless to say, cost goes up significantly as the number of plans within the system, and particularly within an individual insurance carrier, grows. The more plans an individual carrier has, the greater the infrastructure necessary to manage those plans. This means additional staff, training of that staff, additional and more complex information technology, and more variables posing possible "confusion of benefits." Most often the "customer service representative," a non health-care provider, is unaware of the variances among policies, regions, etc. They only know their computer screen. This results in ongoing coverage discrepancies, anger, lost time, and increased health-care expenditures due to the paper shuffle. It does not improve health care. On the backside, or claims processing side of the insurance industry, similar problems are created. One plan covers procedure, but the next does not. Again, more time, more information technology wasted, and so on. All this results in increased cost to all.

In the managed care environment, the managed care company never meets the patient, yet they propel themselves into the role of decision maker about someone's health and well-being. Physicians and other health-care providers have to spend a great deal of time attempting to educate the insurance carrier about why they are making the medical recommendations they are making. This frequently comes in the form of telephone calls, paperwork submission, etc. This is not merely sharing information with the insurance carrier. In essence, the physicians and health-care providers have to "teach" the insurance carrier. In other words, it is like putting them through medical school. Health-care providers often have to say the correct "buzz" words to get procedures approved. It becomes a cat and mouse game. The time spent cannot be recouped directly by doctors, hospitals, and other health-care providers. Hence, this "downtime" results in the provider having to charge more for other services to offset these losses. The provider cannot recoup appropriate reimbursement for their time and expertise. In short, it is managed cost not managed care. The insurance industry is managing money and paper rather than patient care and overall health. They attempt to make decisions based upon incomplete information and from a profit and loss perspective and not a health perspective.

The health insurance industry and the free market system suggests that multiple insurance companies in a for-profit environment fosters better care and lower costs. *Wrong!* First, look at your own health insurance plan and compare it with others. If you compare apples to apples, the cost is essentially the same. Differences in cost are only brought about by Madison Avenue tricks such as the old "bait and switch," the "loss leader," and the old "buy one get one free." Each insurance company lures the consumer in by a sophisticated process conceived in the offices of a Madison Avenue advertising agency. You know what I am saying. They attempt to appeal only to your superficial needs and attempt to set yours apart. In our ever-growing senior sector, the insurance carrier invites our senior citizens to the community country buffet for the "information session." They tell them their plan has an unmatched prescription benefit and they will no longer have to worry about the high cost of medication. It is only after they are signed up and are home reading the fine print that they find the policy caps are a thousand dollars per year and their drugs are not on the insurance carriers' formulary. Yes, that all-important formulary. The magic list of medications that the insurance company struck a deal with the pharmaceutical company for the low rate.

Another company will entice the consumer with a smorgasbord of "preventive" services. These might include a yearly physical, Pap smears, mammograms, prostate or colon screenings, etc. Each of these medical services is excellent to have; but to offset cost, the insurance carrier must limit other services via exclusion, capitation, high deductibles, etc. The insurance company wants to make a sale and subsequent profit. Therefore, they must "hook" the consumer into a particular plan. Again, think of your own health-care plan. When you were confronted with choosing a plan, you typically chose the one that you felt would best meet your needs. That might have been the lower cost for those who have cost as the highest priority. Others might have chosen it for the preventative benefits. You just wanted to know that yearly Pap smear and mammogram were covered because cancer runs in your family. Still others chose it for the prescription benefit due to the need for chronic medication use. Everyone has an agenda of what they *think* they need. Unfortunately, the human body and experience rarely, if ever, allows us to gaze into the crystal ball to predict future needs.

When a person chooses the "wrong" plan or caps are reached in coverage, health care needs continue to march on. What occurs in the American health-care system is the cost of the care begins to get shifted. Usually that cost in some way is shifted to the rest of society. This occurs via accessing health care through inefficient and costly methods such as the emergency room. Most people are not even aware that emergency rooms are required to treat all those who present themselves for care, regardless of their ability to pay. Another scenario exists when an insured person has only a catastrophic plan or a plan that does not cover a particular procedure. What happens then? The same thing that happens at Walmart when somebody shoplifts an item. The cost is shifted to a higher price for all other items to absorb the shoplifting cost.

Our caring, compassionate American society finds a way for individuals to get the health care they need. In over twenty-nine years of working in health care, it finds a way for individuals to get the care they need. It may be inefficient, basic, and so forth but we do not throw people out like some third world countries. The American public would find it unethical and immoral to deny care to someone in need of care. This is not to say that it has never happened or that the business of health care doesn't attempt to pass the buck and defer treatment until absolutely necessary. This occurs and almost always results in higher cost to all. Of course, as is always the case, particularly in the twenty-first century America, the payer of last resort is big brother, the government. Those in need are not turned away. Some federal, state, or other governmental entity steps in and pays for the care. In other words, you and I pay for it.

Beyond the choosing of a health-care plan, there is also the whole issue of the nonprofit and for-profit insurance carrier. Seems simple on the surface, but what a difference. The for-profit insurance carrier must go well beyond just covering cost. It must show a profit to those shareholders who have invested in the company. Since illness does not discriminate between for-profit and nonprofit, the companies themselves must find a way to get a profit. This can only occur through cutting costs, denying service, limiting coverage, and the like. They must attempt to get the care and cost off their back and on the back of someone else…us! Again, the cost-shifting occurs.

The nonprofit on the other hand can take monies and reinvest it into their infrastructure and benefits. This might include additional staff, technology, and benefits. Of course the nonprofit carrier also has costs, but it is not cost-plus profit. The nonprofit is not beholden to shareholders. Furthermore, like most entities, nonprofits can be manipulated as well. They obtain nonprofit status and then pay CEOs, staff, and so forth outrageous sums of money.

Denial of services to the insured is the way for-profit insurance companies attempt to manage cost and promote profit. Even in the case of a policy that is supposed to provide coverage for a certain procedure or diagnosis, countless obstacles are placed in the way of the patient and providers in order to increase cash flow. Imagine delaying approval of the heart bypass surgery or payment on that claim. Now multiply that number by hundreds or even thousands of dollars in deferred or denied payment. Millions of dollars are made in interest investment alone. Welcome to the insurance industry game.

Providers, particularly physicians, are frequently caught between a rock and a hard place in today's health-care environment. In order to survive, physicians have been forced to jeopardize provider contracts, forego referrals, and lose patients. If physicians want to stay in the game, they are squeezed to play within the limitations imposed by the insurance industry. The insurance industry dictates how they will practice or they won't be allowed to participate in the game. Many say that physicians, hospitals, and the like can choose not to accept the rules of the insurance industry; but without the insurance industry, essentially all hospitals, physicians, and health-care providers would be forced out as the average American cannot afford health care of any magnitude without substantial help from the insurance industry. Providers want to continue to practice but are continually struggling with ethics, financial considerations, helping the patient, doing no harm, and so on. The new Hippocratic oath is forced to read, "Thou shalt do no harm unless it costs too much."

CHAPTER 2

Managed Care versus Managed Cost

In chapter 1, I briefly touched on the idea of managed care versus managed cost. There is unequivocally no such thing as managed care. It is an illusion dreamed up by the insurance industry and meetings in the advertising agency offices of Madison Avenue. There is no credible literature that has shown that the management of care from a desk at your insurance company by a "case manager" has resulted in better care than is provided by health-care providers directly involved in the administration of such care.

We have all heard of it or experienced it ourselves. You are admitted to the hospital in California for an appendectomy, and you or hospital personnel must call the insurance carrier in New York to obtain "preauthorization." The case management nurse inevitably states, "I need more information." It is all part of the game between patient, provider, and insurance carrier. If all the t's and i's are not crossed and dotted, it is a convenient loophole to delay or deny "authorization" and subsequent payment. That case manager in New York also doesn't work for free, so there is another layer of bureaucracy with added cost in the provision of care. These are costs that are not necessary to the provision of services but yet add costs to the premiums paid by consumers. Furthermore, the case manager often gets between the patient and health-care provider, often driving a wedge between the two. This often disrupts the provider/patient relationship and interferes with treatment. Additionally, almost always that case manager has never met the patient. In essence, they are practicing medicine, long distance, without meeting the patient, have less training than the provider, and rely heavily on the written word and not the expertise of the treating provider(s). The provider must have a PhD in English and be a good writer rather than an MD focused on care and potentially saving lives.

Insurance industry proponents will argue that they are wanting to make sure the best care possible is made available to the patient. They will even throw out pseudostudies about how their case management program "helps" patient outcomes. What a croc! If nothing else is accomplished in this book, it is hoped that I get people to think. Use the data of one's own life experience. Statistics, studies, and the like have become only substitutes and tools of manipulation around one of the best human tools—*common sense!* Remember, their real agenda is cost, not care. They attempt to make decisions, oftentimes life-threatening, without ever meeting the patient and knowing the whole story. Even when they attempt to get the whole story, this requires time and energy by providers to others who do not know, nor do they care, about the individual. Their allegiance is to the insurance carrier and the bottom line.

Communication between health-care professionals and the insurance carrier is often via telephone, a form, email, or fax. It is impersonal and always incomplete. Medicine does not fit into the pigeonholes of the insurance industry. Each individual patient is unique with their own history, personality, life circumstances, and so forth. You cannot put a square peg in a round hole. That is frequently why medicine is called an art, not a science. Health care is more than beating hearts, bones, muscles, and psyche. It is people.

Medicine does not fit into pigeonholes nor is it mechanistic. There can and should be general guidelines about service provision but each case is unique. Treatment and recovery can be very different from one patient to the next. Some people may have a cold for two days, while others have it for two weeks. The insurance industry, including insurance brought to you by Uncle Sam, Medicare, and Medicaid, has asked for exactness where it is not possible. An appendectomy patient may have three days of recovery approved for a hospital stay; but if the patient requires five days of recovery, the insurance company is off the hook for the cost in many instances. The patient is either sent home prematurely, inviting complications and, therefore, more cost, or they stay for the five days and the cost are deferred to others. Again, increased cost to all. Of course, there are averages, usual circumstances, and typical outcomes. However, only one variable can change the whole scenario.

Your government has taken this problem to new heights with the Medicare program. They developed one of the first "capitated" plans of reimbursement known as Diagnostic-Related Groups (DRGs). This is whereby the government has predetermined what a particular illness or procedure are paid based on that predetermined amount. Uncle Sam was the first to have a crystal ball in this area but not the last. In other words, if Uncle Sam and Medicare believe reasonable reimbursement for an appendectomy is X, then that is what they pay. This is regardless of individual circumstances. They argue that reimbursement is based on averages and it should all come out in the wash. Should unforeseen needs surface, the providers, hospitals, etc. are expected to eat the costs because they did not have the same access to the magic crystal ball that tells what the future individual health-care needs will be. To survive providers, hospitals, and the like are forced to decide between ethics and survival of themselves. This may be through additional DRGs created and manipulation of the system, complications, and a rolling of the dice.

A modification of the DRG system is the commercial capitation plan. Capitation is paying a provider or hospital for care before it is needed. It too is based on statistical averages. Capitation clearly does not work. In the capitated system, the insurance industry can much more accurately predict future cost because care has been prepaid. The providers are saddled with taking all the risk. The system then incents the provider-based prepayment, and the provider is placed in a situation where ethics and morals are again tested to the limit. The formula is simple for the provider. The less you see a patient or the less care/cost incurred, the more that is left over in the end. In this system, the doctor, hospital, or health-care entity quickly learns to cut corners to survive. The short end of the stick goes to the patient and back to society who must incur excessive cost not accounted for in the capitated arrangement. The provider and not the insurance company assumes all the risks. The risks, however, are not in the providers' control. A physician who gets a higher-risk population is at a disadvantage because those patients will require more care. The provider is then caught between the ethical and financial rocks. Not a place where anyone wants to be. Most frequently, providers cannot survive such a system. Health care cannot be solely a business model. It must include the human mode as well.

Insurance companies developed the managed care model about the same time as there was a rise in for-profit insurance companies. They found that they needed a gatekeeper between them the provider and the patient/consumer. They quickly realized the consumer welcomed the case manager because they were convinced, via the insurance company, that they would facilitate care. They would do all this while never eyeballing the patient. The goal is to interfere with the provider/patient relationship, placing doubt and interfering in the trust provided by the provider, an intangible part of medicine.

CHAPTER 3

Government Regulation versus Payment

S hould the government continue to play insurance company? Should they only be in the position of oversight? Maybe they shouldn't be involved in health care at all. Without a doubt health care needs some type of oversight. This is true for a number of reasons. There needs to be regulation of the health insurance industry so that it might be kept orderly, minimally bureaucratic, and honest so that all parties are assured that appropriate care can be afforded to people. Since health care will touch us all, it does seem fitting that the government might best accomplish this objective. After all, in American society, it is looked upon as the entity entrusted with this task. An argument can be made of whether or not that should be the case.

Current examples of where more appropriate oversight is needed are Kaiser Permanente and UnitedHealthCare and their Evercare product. In each of these scenarios, the insurance company also employs the provider. As mentioned earlier, for-profit companies are the proverbial fox guarding the henhouse. While possibly well intentioned, and even put on paper as separate entities, the providers of these carriers, and others like them, employ the very providers entrusted to provide unbiased health care. Pressures are placed on the providers to keep cost down, not to order too many tests, and keep costly procedures to a minimum. The pressure can be undaunting.

The objectivity of the provider is lost when your boss is one of the largest health-care insurers in the country. Implicit and often explicit directives come from above to contain costs or find another job. The provider always knows best but are they allowed to practice based on that knowledge? Not enough safeguards are in place to assure that this will occur. One simple safeguard is not to allow such a grievous conflict of interest.

Oversight is reasonable but regulations have gotten the best of all health care, thereby driving up the cost of care. This ranges from the process of credentialing providers and hospitals to the monsters known as the Health Insurance Portability and Accountability Act (HIPPA) and the Americans with Disability Act (ADA).

The bureaucracy of health care has become its own worst enemy. Take what should be a simple process of becoming a credentialed provider with Medicare. The process is so cumbersome that an individual provider must supply the diploma of the school they graduated from before they can get credentialed. This is in spite of the fact that they must also have to provide Medicare with a copy of their license. Seems reasonable right? Well, what is so ridiculous is that if a provider doesn't have a copy of their diploma, they must get it or not become a provider. Of course, in order to get a license, they obviously must have graduated from the appropriate institution or they would not have been granted the license (issued by an appropriate government agency) they also must produce. This is just a small example, multiplied by many hundreds of times. This leads to lost time and increased cost.

This is but a small example of the hoops that must be jumped. There is no common credential process, no universal form, nothing. With each hospital affiliation, insurance company panel, another form, another layer of bureaucracy. To show you the lunacy found in the Medicare system, they only recently imposed that if a provider needs to notify them of an address change to their practice, they must complete an entire new application. It is over twenty-five pages long! Common sense, a lost concept, would suggest that such a change would be less than a half page in length!

These issues don't hold a candle to HIPPA, a document that reads like a phone book that has led to the creation of countless hours of policy and procedure writing and rewriting. It is a whole new industry within health-care law, and as a good friend of mine who is a health-care attorney says, "It is the attorneys' full employment act." Thousands of pages misinterpreted and misused—all in an attempt to subvert common sense. This act essentially tells the health-care community what it can and cannot do with respect to health-care information, communication, and confidentiality. It is nonsense. I have walked into health-care facilities where the medical charts are now housed in the facility's version of Fort Knox in order to protect privacy. This is necessitated by the fact that a passerby at a nursing station might see the name of a patient on the spine of a chart. We wouldn't want that to happen. Yet, on the same unit, it's okay to place the name of the patient outside their room door. What stupidity! Another example is that a rehabilitation nurse cannot place a sign above a patient's bed indicating that the patient cannot have thin liquids due to a risk of aspiration. Instead, they have to go through a crazy system of "coding" (e.g., the blue dot on the wall means the patient takes nothing by mouth) it so other staff know the patient's needs. Unfortunately, visitors, janitors, and the like do not know the meaning. Like they really care. These hoops lead to mistakes, poor care, increased cost, and even loss of life. That eventually leads to a lawsuit by an attorney looking to line their pockets because of bureaucracy. All these problems are intertwined in the fabric of American health care and have led to the system being broken. One event quickly leads to a chain of events.

Have you ever been admitted to a hospital with some significant illness or disease? I'm sure your only reason for being there was so that you could eavesdrop on your roommate and their doctor discussing that patient's bowel movements. When I have been a patient, I was just worried about getting out, getting better, and eating something other than plastic hospital food brought to you as leftovers from the airline industry. HIPPA wants to put you in a soundproof room in Siberia. Most people don't care about the bowel movements or other physiological happenings of their fellow patients. It most likely will not be the lead story in the *National Enquirer*.

These steps are nothing compared with the steps one professional needs to go through to talk to another professional. It reminds me of the old saying of "I'll have my people talk to your people and we will set something up." That setting something up is usually an act of God! All the time bureaucracy is occurring, time is passing, the meter is running, and the patient is ill and just wants to get better. Yes, to talk to the professional, you better have a release in triplicate and have an attorney on retainer to make sure the writing is HIPPA-compliant or risk a lawsuit because you didn't have the forthwith in the right place.

Such nonsense occurs throughout health care. Have you ever been in line at your local pharmacy waiting for a medication and the sign says, "Do not step in front of this line as it will impinge on the privacy of the person in front of you"? Do you really care that they are purchasing Preparation H? Stupid! Also, when you are in the hospital and your physician comes in to speak with you. He pulls the curtain and commences to discuss your medical case with you. All the time your roommate is in the next bed and that curtain is supposed to stop sound waves from traveling ten feet across the room. Do you think they really care? It is much more likely they are just worried about getting out of the hospital themselves.

Another ingenious brainchild of lawyers was the Americans with Disabilities Act (ADA), a second document rivaling that of HIPPA and the Bible in length. Unlike the Bible but similar to HIPPA, it is hundreds of pages to explain common sense. While I am the first to admit that common sense has come to be lacking in the mush of America, a document attempting to legislate it will not bring it back and only serves to impede care, dignity, and compassion. Attorneys looking to file frivolous lawsuits and go onto the *Talking Heads* television shows love it. Remember it guarantees the full employment of your local attorney. A small faction of society makes the decisions for the greater whole.

Regulation should be narrow in focus and limited to care. Your government should also remove itself from the role of insurance payer. One should always do what one is best at doing. The government's best role is not of insurance carrier/payer. Since 1963 and Lyndon Johnson's Great Society, countless billions have been spent on government-sponsored health care through Medicare, Medicaid, and other indigent programs. It has led to government waste, corruption, bureaucracy, and expansion into individual American lives.

Programs such as Medicare and Medicaid find themselves so filled with the burden of red tape and regulation that they routinely have another arm of government, the Office of the Inspector General, seek out and pursue hospitals and providers for improper provision of care and subsequent reimbursement based on thousands of pages of rules and regulations rivaling that of the US tax code. Should a provider "step out of bounds," they are threatened with fines, criminal prosecution, disenrollment, and so forth. The government then feels very proud of itself in "catching" these providers who had no intent of not following the rules but rather those who didn't know the rule/regulation existed or where it contradicts itself in its own regulations. These are not the bad eggs found in every profession/industry. This is the provider or hospital that had to be more worried about the bulletin that was published with the latest bureaucratic change rather than taking care of their patients. Daily, this drives excellent providers from the ranks of health care into anything but the paper-driven, endless cycle of treating the paper and regulation as the patient. The very reason most entered health care was to help their fellow man in need. In what other profession are there regulations such that you can go back seven years and request recoupment of reimbursement of services? Would you want to have such a work environment? As a plumber, if a customer came back seven years later and said I want my money back because I don't really think I needed that new pipe, what would you think? Would you see it as fair? Reasonable? Or ridiculous? These are the regulations, guidelines, and bureaucracy providers must contend with and still provide good care.

Even the reimbursement and claims process is a cesspool of paper, added time, cost, and complexity. Can you imagine the number of steps and stops a claim must take just to get it paid? Needless steps and middlemen. Usually, the patient just thinks I have insurance and my doctor or hospital will take care of it. From the minute you hand over your insurance card, the gears begin to turn with countless steps before payment is received. You must present your card, and the insurance must be verified and possibly preauthorized. You are then seen and treated, and a charge is created. This is accomplished by a form or two or three. It is sent to coding, then to the billing office. At the billing office, all your demographic information is entered, the procedure code, diagnosis code, place of service, provider number, etc. You would then think it would be whisked away via technology to the insurance company. No. No. The claim then goes to a clearinghouse to assure formatting is correct. From the clearinghouse it goes to the insurance company. At that point, it must be received in the correct claims department for the correct plan. Remember, your insurance company may have twenty, thirty, forty different plans to administer, each with its own nuances. Once processed then reimbursement is authorized and it goes back to the provider. This is the case only if it is a "clean" claim. Any problems with the claim may switch it to a totally manual system that may result in the claim having to be resubmitted all over again. This may take weeks, sometimes months. All the time your doctor gets reluctant to see you again because your insurance company is not paying its claims. This sometimes to get a twenty-dollar check. The process can be quite cumbersome, inefficient, antiquated, and quite troubling for provider and payer alike.

Can you imagine Mastercard, Visa, or American Express operating in such a fashion? The last time I checked, I was in and out at a checkout counter in a store after running my credit card in less than a minute. When was the last time your statement was messed up through one of these companies?

Waste is prolific in the health insurance industry. Uncle Sam, the insurance carrier (e.g., Medicaid), is so riddled with bureaucracy they will send the same monthly bulletin to each provider in a group, each month, even though that group submits claims under one provider number. In our group alone with twenty-three providers at forty-one cents per bulletin, per month, plus printing costs. Each and every month. The most laughable part is that we get ten additional bulletins each month for providers that haven't been with our group for many years. Some are even dead. This is in spite of telephone conversations requesting it be stopped and written correspondence with *their* forms, and it still doesn't stop. If people don't think those nickels and dimes don't add up...give them all to me.

Approximately 48 percent of every health-care dollar is spent to pay for bureaucracy and not for direct health care. Middleman after middleman. Electronic billing, billing offices, clearinghouses, case managers, preauthorization, rebilling, contract negotiation, needless and useless documentation, defensive medicine, malpractice insurance, front office people, and back-office people. The list is endless. Attempts must be made to eliminate waste in bureaucracy not care. Even eliminating 1 percent of this could save the system an estimated three billion dollars per year.

CHAPTER 4

MD versus MBA
Is Your Doctor Corporate America?

D o you want your local MBA or bean counter making your diagnosis and determining your treatment? Well, it happens every day. The infiltration of corporate America and "big business" has led to medical decisions being made based on profit rather than medical need. Shareholders and CEOs make the decisions, not surgeons and internists. Columbia Healthcare, the nation's largest health-care corporation, founded by Richard Scott promised us the best health care for the lowest price. Has this happened? No. Go to any Columbia Healthcare hospital, or for that matter any for-profit hospital, and the cost of an appendectomy, bypass surgery, or newborn delivery will be essentially the same. The difference is that the for-profit health-care facilities must show a profit and be able to provide the shareholders with a dividend check or face loss of company value and market share. The nonprofit institution reinvests via new equipment, more staff, better staff, and expansion of services.

The administration and management of corporate health care are making decisions directly affecting medical outcomes based solely on the perceived bottom line. I say perceived because their decisions often make a quarterly report look better; but the intangibles of increased litigation, staff turnover, community reputation, etc. are difficult to measure in dollars and cents. Institutional medicine is now managed like Walmart. The patient is the commodity, and you are frequently felt to be expendable. Would you go to your doctor to have him or her tell you what engine to put in your car or what the problem is with your plumbing? Of course not. Then why should an MBA decide on what your medical treatment should be?

Since the advent of corporate medicine, people who are patients have now become nothing more than customers, consumers, and a demographic to have the latest sales pitch thrown at them. People, who unfortunately become patients, something we all will experience at some time, are not a consumer at your local Walmart or big-box store looking to buy a refrigerator with the most bells and whistles for the lowest price. They are individuals forced into a system of immense complexity, requiring unmatched trust and often-blind faith. It is a system that says, "I'm sick. I need help." It is to such an extent it literally may become a life-and-death situation. It is a system of forced choice of entry. Almost no one wants to go see a doctor. You don't get to pick an illness. You would rather be anywhere else. The evolution of the health-care system has tried to suggest it is some-thing other than a forced choice.

The marketing of health-care plans, hospitals, pharmaceuticals, and the like is not about good health care or the provision of infor-mation; it is about the sale and the dollars, cosmetically concealed to such an extent that even a Beverly Hills plastic surgeon would be envious. What is there to market? You only get one body. You can't trade it in and get the new model. Prior to Madison Avenue's make-over of health care and the onslaught of big profit medicine, you didn't have to have your doctor or hospital advertise. You knew where they were and how to get there if you *needed* them. Marketing costs attempt to sell and bring in more revenue. Therefore, if no advertis-ing were evident, health-care costs would diminish.

Without a doubt the health insurance industry, pharmaceutical industry, and your local investment group solicits illness. The health insurance industry markets multiple plans each with their individual enticements. Low deductibles, "free" physicals, preventive medicine, no preauthorization, and so on all attempt to lure the patient, seen as a customer, to the low price, best product, etc. The permutations of these loss leaders are endless. What happens when you pick the plan and then it doesn't have the coverage you need? You access treatment only to find bureaucracy, anxiety, headaches, and the corporate "soft-shoe." You must get treatment and then find another way to get it paid for. Often the cost is passed through the system eventually landing back on other individuals and not the company that sold you that wonderful policy in the first place.

The pharmaceutical industry has also made an appealing splash. You know the ones I mean. The "Purple Pill" or that antidepressant ad that features the highly attractive thirty-year-old female who is now on top of the world because of Zoloft, or Prozac, or Paxil, or whatever new cocktail professing to be a panacea is what they are hawking. You didn't even know you were depressed until you saw the commercial and you were missing out on the "good life." Now you are depressed because you haven't been taking an antidepressant, the magic pill. But you are advised to fix it by going to your doctor to discuss your needs. The commercial was so helpful that it even tells you what the doctor needs to give you. Why bother with medical school? You can just provide a menu to your patient and phone in the order. The United States by far expends far more money on medication than any other industrialized country.

Additionally, the United States essentially subsidizes the cost of medication in other countries. We frequently pay a much bigger price for the same medicine. Why? Because the pharmaceutical industry has learned that the American public will pay almost anything. Even the government is in on the act. Medicare is not even allowed to negotiate the lowest price for a medication even when competition exists. Another government program gone array. Millions upon millions wasted annually.

Scare tactics are even better to "inform" you of what you need. How about that radio ad in your community that tells you that you better run down and get your heart scan or risk getting up in the morning and not even being able to say good morning to your spouse before a catastrophic heart attack kills you? You have to get a heart scan now even though you have never been sick a day in your life, are thirty years old, run five miles a day, and don't drink or smoke. That investment group that funded that scanner expects to optimize utilization to pay for the millions invested for that scanner. They expect to make a profit, almost entirely based on fear.

Big Pharma and the insurance industry, through lobbying efforts, assure the golden egg via politicians and agencies of power. Knowing the right people at the right time is advantageous to the large health-care corporations looking at bottom-line profits.

It used to be common that your local doctor had his/her own office, sometimes with one or more colleagues. They were told that they did not know business and were inefficient. They were gradually convinced that the others were correct. Furthermore, the front office became more and more bureaucratic. More and more a business model prevailed. Gradually practices were managed by health-care management companies. A middleman is introduced. Practices then went beyond just practice management companies. Hospitals began buying up physician practices. Often this was to exercise control and to better funnel patients to their hospitals. The separation of physicians and hospitals have become nonexistent. As a result, hospital administrations through their implicit pressure and even explicit pressure influence physicians clinically in an effort to keep cost down: less tests, shorter stays, etc. Previously there was a distinct separation between the two, especially from a financial perspective. The clinical judgment is inherently affected. All this change has been insidious and quite frequently not even conscious. Physicians have been convinced that it is simpler. They no longer have to worry about the direct business aspects of a practice. They may also accept a salary from the hospital that owns the practice.

Slowly there has also been the evolution of practices where their physicians never set foot in a hospital. Their practice is limited to outpatient. Should their patient need hospitalization, they are handed off to hospital-based physicians and even hospitalists. Such physicians have no outpatient. In other words, the patient becomes a hot potato. In the prior model, the physician knew their patient from head to toe. When the new inpatient physician takes over control in some ways, they must start from scratch. They do not know the idiosyncrasies of the patients and each of their ins and outs. In the prior model, they knew everything about their patients and would follow them in any setting, hospital, office, nursing home, and the like. Which is better both financially and clinically? Does better clinical management have intangible gains that are difficult to assess and therefore beyond a financial formula?

CHAPTER 5

Profit versus Nonprofit

Insurance companies battle with individuals supposedly insured on what is covered and what is not. If an individual insurance carrier pays for two days in the hospital after childbirth, they will be hard-pressed to pay for a third day even if the individual patient needs it according to their health-care provider. Insurance companies are not in a place to make those decisions. The late time I looked UnitedHealthCare and Aetna did not graduate magna cum laude from their local medical school. Decisions are routinely made from a desk far, far away. The individual insurance company employee who pulls the plug on coverage has never met the individual with the medical need. Certainly, that person never went to medical school.

Mental health services in almost every instance are determined not by need but by a dollar amount or the number of sessions. This determination is not based on any treatment theory, treatment model, or research indicating this is appropriate. The decision is based on cost containment needs. This population of patients, as well as a growing number of our elderly, is those most easily exploited. They do not have the ability or wherewithal to fight the system. Often these mentally or physically impaired individuals don't even have the ability or access to exercise their voice through the vote.

Unlike nonprofit medicine health care, decisions are more likely made based upon shareholder interests and not the individual's needs. Institutional medicine in the for-profit sector will often forego new equipment unless it is a profit center, better staffing, new facilities, and such because the stockholder expects a dividend check. They expect money back on their investment. Companies cut corners in order to maximize profits. This leaves the burden of mediocre to substandard care to that of patients, society, government, and the individual taxpayer.

Whatever an insurance company denies in health care, the cost is then shifted to another sector. It does not just go away. A catastrophic illness may not be covered by an individual policy but the patient does not go untreated. Instead the cost is shifted to another payer source, usually the taxpayer. Mental health benefits may have a yearly maximum of 2,500 dollars. For a patient with major mental illness, this often would not cover the treatment needed. They are still treated; however, it is now through an inefficient manner. The insurance company does not pay for it. The burden goes to the public sector and the taxpayer—morality and ethics superseded by greed. Providers don't allow the patient to die but the provider must often treat the person for free.

Another cost containment technique is that of denying or limiting coverage for preexisting conditions. This is especially true if the diagnosis is a high dollar one. For-profit insurance companies by their very nature want to ensure individuals that are healthy, access health care minimally, and cost the least. In general, that is of course, the young, disease-free, males, higher educational level, higher socioeconomic status, and the like—any demographic that puts them in a group that accesses health care and therefore insurance less often. By excluding higher-risk individuals on any parameter, that increases the statistical probability that they will need health care. The insured sample becomes very skewed and therefore a better risk for the insurance company. After all, *insurance is shared risk*.

A relatively new but quite disturbing concept has been the development and implementation of the insurer/provider model. The insurer and provider are one and the same. Examples include Evercare, a UnitedHealthCare product, Kaiser Permanente, and other companies promoting a capitated model of reimbursement. PacifiCare may pay a physician six dollars/month whether they need to treat the patient or not. The provider is "prepaid." When such a model is the case, treatment is not provided based on need but rather on economics. It is survival of the financially fittest. Cost increases because if treatment is not based on need, additional treatment is necessary. When the insurance carrier employs the provider directly, that is the fox guarding the henhouse. You derive your livelihood from a company that has direct control based on cost rather than need. Deadly results are often seen.

Insurance company managers are rewarded for cost containment and profits rather than the good management of health needs. Such measures result in cost-shifting; but remember, pay me now or pay me later.

Hospitals and insurance companies should not be allowed to exploit and profit from the unfortunate circumstances of another, particularly when they have no control over the illness that confronts them. Unlike almost all commodities, health care is not ruled by purely capitalistic tenets. Sickness and injury almost always dictate entry into the health-care arena. Most often individuals do not have a choice. It is forced upon them. It is also usually an all-or-nothing proposition. In a purely capitalistic system, when one elects to buy a new refrigerator with stainless steel and the ice maker in the door and a budget of $1,500, one can decide to buy or not. If the refrigerator is $2,000, you may have to elect to stay within budget and only get a black one with a regular ice maker. It is voluntary. Having health care thrust upon us is most often not voluntary and is necessity. You don't say when contemplating surgery, "Hey doc, skip the sutures. I want to save $500.00." It is forced and all-or-nothing.

These ads pressure doctors and other providers to dispense medicine based on public pressure not good medicine. Western philosophy is that of the magic pill. The idea is that you should never hurt or have pain. You should be physically and emotionally numb. In other words, patient sees ad and goes to doctor, patient pesters doctor based on misguided or incomplete information, and then doctor is placed in a precarious situation. The doctor wants to help the patient and keep them under their care; but if they say no to the patient, they risk the patient, which then becomes a doctor shopper. Good medicine is between the patient and the physician. The advertising executive should not be in the examination room.

The Madison Avenue Medical School practices medicine every day. Any advertisement leads the medical community to practice medicine in a certain way. Ads are constructed to sell medicine, not promote health. Packaging; the presentation of the everyday person with upset stomachs, headaches, diarrhea, and countless other ailments; and catchy wording grab even the most cautious individual in their web. Even the providers get bombarded with free pens, clipboards, free dinners, and other perks to sell medicine. This leads to pressure on the provider to use a medicine, not because it is needed or the best, but because they feel guilty because of the expensive dinner they had last night provided by the medicine's manufacturer.

CHAPTER 6

Madison Avenue versus
the Hippocratic Oath

You have all seen or heard it. You know—the "purple pill." "Are you sad…" The Hippocratic oath has taken a back seat to Madison Avenue and corporate profit. America is looking for the magic pill, and the largest of the New York advertising firms and the pharmaceutical industry are more than happy to provide it. You see it on your television every day. The young healthy blonde female who is no longer depressed because of the latest and greatest antidepressant, or Ambien, promising that full night's sleep. Then there are those statin drugs alluding to heading off that heart attack or stroke. Why I'm not taking them? I better talk to my doctor right away. After all I'm a time bomb waiting to go off. The thirty-second television spot immediately surpasses four years of medical school and three to seven years of residency training. The slick packaging of the television or radio commercial or even print ad provides the patient, or as the advertising firm would have it the "consumer," with the perfect opportunity to exploit the vulnerable, suggestible, often terrified patient with the magic cure. All that without even having to go to the doctor's office.

The United States has 5 percent of the world's population, yet it consumes 70 percent of the world's prescribed medication. Phenomenal numbers wouldn't you say? Phenomenal but true. The last time I looked, I don't think we were the sickest population on the planet. I thought we had advanced knowledge, medicine, and science. Oh, but I forgot our most advanced discipline is advertising and hype.

The manufacturers of the drugs go through all their silly disclaimers mandated by Uncle Sam only to promise you the moon. Of course, they say they are only "educating" the public and the public has the "right to know." Hogwash! Education and decisions about treatment alternatives are *solely* a function of the doctor/patient relationship. Madison Avenue has no place in the examination room. The doctor and the patient should not have the influence of finely crafted advertising. The patient sees or hears an ad and then talks with the doctor who may say no. Often this results in the patient losing confidence in the doctor because they have been unduly influenced by advertisement telling them that they *need* that pill. If the physician or provider does not give in, the patient then simply doctor shops until they hear what they want to hear. It is implied that the advertiser of drug is correct and they know what you need and the doctor does not.

The practitioner is then placed in a precarious position: prescribe the pill or risk losing a patient to doctor shopping, resulting in loss of livelihood, or prescribe it and risk the practice of compromised medicine. The physician then thinks, "Well, if I prescribe it, I can at least keep an eye on my patient."

Advertising doesn't stop with medication. Durable medical equipment is just as prone to the direct advertising. It may be the scooter chair, "Hurricane," catheters, or even prosthesis for hip replacement. Pressure is then placed upon the doctor to prescribe the medical equipment or risk alienating a patient and even losing them if you do not succumb to their wishes. Companies insist that they are only educating the public and patients. This supposedly occurs in a one-minute commercial, one-page ad, or a radio spot. Can you imagine a patient going to see his orthopedic surgeon before hip surgery and asking, "What type of hip prosthesis are you using? I saw a commercial with Arnold Palmer, and he recommends *Stryker*. I only want *Stryker*. I don't want any of that Ace Hardware stuff!" The patient would not know one prosthesis from another.

As mentioned earlier the use of advertising provides misguided and slanted information to the individual patient and society as a whole. Ads for the multibillion-dollar pharmaceutical industry imply a lack of normalcy if you don't use their pill. You might be eighty years old with normal aches and pains, but the industry implies the magic pill provides the fountain of youth. A thirty-second ad, or a one-paragraph ad, replaces years of medical training and thousands of patient hours for what medicine should be used, when they should be used, drug interactions, diagnoses, and so on.

Each television or radio advertisement and each print ad in your favorite magazine increases the cost of your health care. The marketers of these medications, therapies, treatments, diagnostic tests, and the like will tell you that it is for your education and you have the right to know and the right of choice. A little truth can be a dangerous thing especially to Americans who are in constant search for the fountain of youth and that magic pill. If we only had a pill to cure gullibility!

Advertisement and marketing do not stop at the patients' front door. It hits the health-care providers as well. It comes in the form of pens, paper, travel bags, dinners, junkets, "training seminars," and so forth. The bottom line is using our product. The manufacturers and "reps" as they are most often referred to are highly trained, highly paid and used car salespeople. They have very polished presentations and expense budgets that are second to none. I have had the opportunity to play the role of "educator" with one of the largest pharmaceutical companies in the nation. They supply the slides and the studies that support the use of their medication or profit, and quite frequently they even fund the studies. No conflict, there right? I stopped this practice, as I was not allowed to truly entertain the audience's real questions. It was all quite staged. My ethics said no. It only presented the good side of the apple. The providers were not allowed to really see the wormhole on the backside. Many very reputable providers get sucked in, however. After all, the perks are quite enticing. I personally was paid over $1500.00/hour plus expenses. Believe me, I didn't have to eat at Taco Bell.

Somebody has to pay for all this provision of "information." The manufacturers have to recoup these expenditures. This increases the cost well beyond the initial cost for the research and development of the drug, durable medical equipment/device, or the procedure. Money expended must be recouped vis-a-vis the product they are pitching. These companies don't spend money because they are a bunch of altruistic nice guys from lower Manhattan. It is passed on to the system via higher insurance premiums, higher health-care costs, etc. They don't plan on losing money on the investment. They will market the drug, procedure, gadget, or whatever to recoup and make a profit even when the market is not there. They will create a market.

One of my favorite areas of health-care advertisement is that of marketing your local hospital. Don't you already know where your local hospital is located? Today, hospitals are "forced" to market to keep themselves financially solvent. Or so they say. Most hospitals are marketed more effectively than the Four Seasons. Many even come with a pool, fireplace, dinner dining on white linen, and even an after-dinner drink. You think I'm kidding. Go see your local hospital and see what it has to offer. Be especially interested in the tour of the for-profit ones.

It doesn't stop with hospitals. Have you heard your local radio station ad for the "heart scan?" Yes, they now scare you to death basically implying that if you do not get your heart scan before midnight tonight, the ticking time bomb inside you will go off. Ron Popeil would be proud of that advertising strategy. Unfortunately, investor groups have gotten a hold of invaluable technology and corrupted its use through scare tactics. But guess what—they are laughing all the way to the bank!

CHAPTER 7

Efficient versus Inefficient Health Care

Many studies and surveys have suggested that as many as forty million Americans are without health insurance. First, I contend that number is usually banted about by the scaremongers in favor of Hillary's plan for socialized medicine or as her package would suggest, "universal health care." We already have universal health care. We just don't have universal payment or an efficient delivery system. In almost twenty-nine years of working in health care, I have yet to see a person go untreated. This includes the intercity hospitals of Chicago to the private practices of the suburbs. People get treatment. Unfortunately, it is frequently provided in the most inefficient and costly settings.

When people do not have a true health-care plan, they most often access health care at the most expensive point of entry, the emergency room. Why? Well, frequently, they wait because they don't want to expend personal resources for care. They would sooner have a second car, new TV, bigger house, or some other personal item. They are *entitled* to care.

Another reason often accessed, particularly by system-savvy individuals, is the fact that thanks to big brother an emergency room cannot turn somebody away for their inability to pay. The EMTALA statute does not allow those individuals who present to an emergency room to be turned away regardless of ability to pay or country of origin (I'll address this crisis later).

The American public has learned not to wait. If I can't get a doctor's appointment, I will go to the emergency room. This becomes an abuse to the system. Insurance companies have tried to curtail this practice by implementing a surcharge if it is determined not to be an emergency. The provider system has compensated for this by making everything an emergency if that is what it takes to get paid. Who are we fooling? The current system is set up for people to migrate to the most inefficient and costly point of entry. The incentives are not to stay healthy and nip it in the bud.

One of my favorite fallacies in the health-care system is that of the repetitive, perfunctory paperwork. The "system" has attempted to endorse and propagate the silly notion of "If it isn't on paper, it didn't happen." Essentially every health-care worker, from orderly to physician, has that drilled into his or her heads. What a joke. Do you actually believe that just because it is on paper it did happen? When I entered the health-care field some twenty-nine years ago, the documentation that was completed was done in order to communicate between professionals. Today, that is but a secondary or even tertiary reason to document. Now the primary reason for documentation is to keep some bureaucrat happy at some governmental agency or some far removed insurance company. It has nothing to do with quality health care. Documentation used to occur by exception. In other words, you wrote something down if it was of significance to the care of the patient. Today, you have to write, "The patient is okay… The patient is stable…" You are required to state the obvious.

Paperwork and this mentality are born out of mistrust. Those who endorse this methodology of "a note for every charge" are quite naive. It gives the reader, often a payer source, a false sense of security. That is the mentality that writing it down makes it so. Health care providers have "learned" the system, and the information is manipulated to meet the needs of the writer or to pacify the system rather than to improve the health of the patient. This occurs even though the information may not be accurate or true. It is done to try to get care for the patient and have a successful outcome. The bottom line is the paper is the patient. The patient is not the patient. To succeed in health care, don't go to medical school and get an MD or nursing school to get an RN or BSN. Go to college and get a PhD in English. If you are a good writer, no matter how poor of a provider you are, you will do well.

Once upon a time, when I was a Boy Scout, their oath started with the words "A scout is trustworthy, loyal…" In today's health-care environment there is no trust. Insurers don't trust providers, patients don't trust insurers, providers don't trust insurers, and on and on. Trust is a necessary but intangible aspect of good health care. By trying to turn medicine into a mechanistic process, costs increase. If trust was part of the equation, cost could be cut. Unfortunately, the lack of trust in others is not limited to health care in America. The level of distrust itself is contagious and has been an ever-increasing cancer in American society. No trust in your fellow man. Health care providers have found that a third party, the insurer, has become the patient. The provider must justify treatment, diagnosis, etc. to the company rather than to the patient. The system then stagnates and cannot move forward.

The lack of trust leads to increased stress on the system, increased costs, and bureaucracy, which take valuable resources away from patient care. One example is the tension created between the insurer and the provider, resulting in the patient getting caught in the middle. This increased stress in the patient which can exacerbate symptoms and increase treatment and recovery time. All this leads to animosity and increased financial costs.

Utilization review initiated by the insurance carrier is another venue of distrust. By definition, utilization review by the insurer suggests that there is the possibility that the provider is doing something wrong or unnecessary. A business entity in essence is called upon to make medical decisions. Insurance carriers like to say they have case managers to enhance treatment, but they are nothing less than gatekeepers, hired for the specific purpose to police the providers. This creates immediate mistrust and an explicit or implicit adversarial relationship. The needless time and money spent on these aspects takes away from the real business of caring for those who are ill.

Contrary to the American desire for the very clean scientific model, the system cannot operate efficiently or satisfactorily without trust. While not tangible, without it the system falters. The lack of it leads to more bureaucracy that leads to more costs. The very nature of the current system promotes an us-versus-them mentality.

When I started in health care over two and a half decades ago, medical documentation was for communication between health-care professionals and to provide clinical data to enhance outcomes. Today, documentation is largely a justification provided to a payer source. The medical record should have nothing to do with the payer source. When the medical record becomes justification to a payer source, costs rise and nonmedical people become unnecessarily involved.

Almost half of health-care costs are not care related but rather bureaucracy and paperwork. There is coding, accounting, claims management (providers and insurers), utilization review, case managers, help lines, consumer relations, billing companies, clearinghouses, auditors, fraud departments, and so on. With each of these layers of bureaucracy come salaries, which increase costs. Yet not one of these areas enhances health care or helps to make the patient better.

Health-care providers are more appreciated for being good at English and sentence structure than they are for excellent health care. The fallacy set forth is that good verbiage equates to good health care. Poor verbiage equals a poor provider. The layers of the bureaucracy truly believe the paper is the patient. The paperwork does not portray the therapeutic relationship/alliance and its importance in the health-care process. A simplistic, yet powerful example of this variable was seen in the movie *Doc Hollywood*. In this movie, Michael J. Fox plays an up and coming physician who is sentenced to serve as town physician for destroying the local judge's fence with his car. A scene unfolds with Fox's diagnosis of "mitral valve regurgitation" in a young boy who presents with his parents to the town hospital. He was ready to air evacuate the boy to the big city hospital for this diagnosis, but then the usual town's physician enters the picture and diagnosed the boy with an upset stomach because he had gotten into his parents' homemade remedy for an upset stomach. He took too much and the town physician had encountered this before in the boy. In the end he was treated with a can of *Coke*. Certainly, simplistic in its presentation; but the bottom line is that good old Doc Hogg, the town physician, knew the boy, his family, and his history of getting into mom and dad's things. In the movie's case, it saved the boy from unnecessary open-heart surgery. People say, "Oh that's the movies. Nothing like that happens in real life." It happens every day, unnecessary care due to the lack of a therapeutic relationship with the patient.

Remember the days when you actually knew the doctor's name and who you were working with at any given time. Not true anymore in today's assembly-line medicine. HMOs are the worst in this regard. HMOs such as Kaiser Permanente will often have a patient see a new physician each time they present themselves in the clinic. Better yet, the physicians now have a tribe of nurse practitioners and physician assistants who see the patients as "patient extenders." They increase profit and keep the assembly line moving. Each time the new practitioner is starting from scratch. No real history, rapport, and relationship with the patient. Just the last provider's progress note. Some are detailed; but more often than not, it is "just the facts." There are no qualitative aspects to the intervention. Medicine is as much art as it is science. There is a reason it was referred to as the medical arts. If that were not the case, anyone could be the physician or nurse practitioner, physician's assistant, or what have you.

If you have the same doctor, with whom you have a relationship, he or she gets to *know* you. For example, if Joe comes in and complains of pain, he/she will have some idea as to the legitimacy of the complaint. If the doctor does not know Joe, he/she may order tests, x-rays, and examinations which are not necessary because they didn't know that Joe is just a chronic complainer. This of course can increase cost unnecessarily and protract care. It may also reinforce dependence on the health-care system.

Another major barrier in the current health-care system is that there has been a strong disincentive for providers to communicate with each other. The providers' communication with others is essentially "downtime." Time and knowledge are their expertise. If they are not compensated for it, the provider becomes reluctant to spend a whole lot of time on it. While this communication may significantly shorten a course of treatment or limit intervention, it is often sacrificed due to time or monetary constraints. Providers have been forced to focus on their little slice of the pie. For example, you slip and fall on the weekend, necessitating a trip to the emergency room. The doctor examines you, gets some x-rays, but then concludes it is a muscle pull. He gives you some pain medication and tells you if it still hurts in three days, go see your family doctor. You are still in pain in three days and you go and see him. What does he do? Examination, x-rays, blood work, etc. All those things you had done in the emergency room. He may do it out of laziness to get the prior records, he may have equipment that must be paid for and tests are a profit center, or he just might not know what was done due to a lack of interaction with the emergency room physician. No matter what costs have gone up, care has not necessarily improved.

Another popular trend in health-care limiting the doctor-patient relationship has been the movement toward segmented care. The hospitalist who is a physician that just sees inpatients or the outpatient physician who treats only clinic patients. Constant compartmentalizing of care. The former model had the physician knowing his or her patient from head to toe. This trend is not only in physician care but in nursing care as well.

Many years ago, nursing was driven by primary nursing. A given nurse was assigned a given number of patients. He/she knew those patients from bedpans, to medication, to skincare, and how old their children were. They knew their patients. Now that is all changed. Today there are "medication" nurses who do nothing but administer medication or "treatment" nurses who provide prescribed treatments. It doesn't stop there. There are restorative nurses responsible for ambulation, IV nurses for starting and monitoring IVs, etc. None of this was implemented for care but for cost containment. It may seem like money was saved but the long-term costs are immeasurable. Nurses largely know nothing about the patients they work with on a day-to-day basis.

Inefficiency also occurs when community resources are lacking. Insurance companies often have designated facilities or hospitals which are often not the closest or most convenient to the patient's proximity. While "costs" may not be directly measured in dollars, they are often measured in care or the lack thereof. A recent example was that endured by my former sister-in-law. She is thirty-nine years old who began suffering from leg pain and pain in her arm and upper chest area. She called the Kaiser office closest to her house (less than five miles) but was told that she needed to go to a Kaiser clinic some twenty-five miles from her home to "have an ultrasound." She followed their instructions. Upon arrival at the clinic twenty-five miles away, she was seen and had an ultrasound done. They suspected a life-threatening pulmonary embolus. As a result, she was then told to go to the Kaiser hospital, another eighteen miles away, for a CAT scan. She was not taken by ambulance even though the emboli could move and almost instantly kill her. Instead she was just given instructions not to drive herself. Luckily, she was able to call my wife who instantly became the local ambulance and emergency medical technician all rolled into one. The resources were all within her own backyard, but she could not use them because it wasn't convenient to the insurance carrier. The cost of her life was on the line to "save" a dollar. Well, how much money, psychological trauma, and the like could have been saved if there was efficiency to see her doctor, in her own community, and go to the hospital in her community, where her doctor is and where the relationship is with her providers and family.

Inefficiency is also found in the day-to-day functions of hospitals, day surgery centers, skilled nursing facilities, and so forth. Nurses in hospitals often spend their valuable time typing progress notes and other forms of documentation. A nurse's salary and skills to be a typist? Certified nursing assistants who spend half a shift or more doing housekeeping. The system believes it is saving money. Instead, it is creating further inefficiency. It also increases the possibility of errors. Shifting skills of a trained person to that of a foreign job duty creates the likelihood of inefficiency by not having an appropriate person completing job duties for which they were trained and have an interest. Furthermore, the lack of personnel such as a ward secretary slows down health care, eliminates a layer of checks and balances, and increases the possibility of clinical errors. In years past this was not the case but corporate medicine tries to get blood out of a turnip.

Finally, there is no centralized database in health care. It is often incomplete, fragmented, and piecemeal. With the transient nature of America and the even more transient nature of constant changes in health plans, employers, providers, and such, valuable information is constantly lost, and "new" data must be reconstructed. We have a centralized database for our financial information but not for something more important than money—our health.

CHAPTER 8

The HIPPA and ADA America's Answer to Illogical Information Sharing and Disabling America

The Healthcare Insurance Portability and Accountability Act (HIPPA) enacted in 1996 has become the second wave of the attorney's full employment act right after America's other disaster, the Americans with Disabilities Act. The implementation of this act rivaling that of our income tax system has only encouraged litigation for infractions, decreases trust, and assumes that "others" really care about your health. Embedded in the very core of HIPPA is the assumption that somebody else really cares about how you are doing medically. There is the paranoia that now "I can get the dirt on him." There is this strong belief that the information will be used against the person. Are we naïve enough to think that if someone wanted to "get us" they would need medical information?

We expend far too much in the way of time, energy, and money to protect a few. A few might get bent out of shape if someone knows about his or her health condition, but at what cost financially and medically? People are far too busy to care what the latest tabloid happens to be about their neighbor. Can you remember the last time you were in the hospital and you wanted to stay longer so that you could find out the diagnosis and tragedy of your hospital roommate?

Do you plan on calling your local news station so it could be the lead story? The people I know were only interested in getting out of the hospital as fast as possible.

The illogic of HIPPA has led to patient charts being locked in a room and even a second chart being created at times because of mental health information being created. This has resulted in the impeded transference of information between professionals, time delays in care, and of course, increased costs. Simple things such as active patient boards in emergency rooms or on patient units had to be removed or covered. Worksheets that might have patient names have to be covered. Patient names are taken from the doors on patient rooms in hospitals. The list goes on and on. It leads to increased time, confusion, and, yes, even life-threatening circumstances. Within the last year, I was personally aware of an instance where a chart was locked up for privacy, and that privacy cost the person their life. The individual was coded (had a heart attack) and the nurse did not know if the patient was full core (all measures taken to revive them). By the time the chart was located and then the information in the chart communicated, the patient had been in code status for an extended period of time. The person may have died anyhow but the protracted time did not help the cause. Was it better to ensure good care or protect the name?

How about those handicapped parking spaces? How many acres of America's real estate are set aside for handicapped parking? Most of it is usually empty. Oh, and by the way, why does a deaf person need a placard for handicapped parking? Does walking less improve hearing? Why is it that if the handicap has nothing to do with ambulation, you need to park closer? By the way, in our world of the politically correct, the people are not handicapped. They are "physically challenged" or "sensory challenged" or what have you. Just the use of these phrases cost my publisher more money in print! Each of these little nuances costs us.

The HIPPA and the ADA have done nothing but make lawyers wealthy. They have created increased divisiveness in society. Instead of doing something for someone who is handicapped or disadvantaged out of empathy or a genuine caring, it is forced upon us by the lawyers and a small fraction of "do-gooders." Rather than building bridges between people, it has generated chasms. The lawyers and big brother have created friction. Generally, people want to do the right thing. Laws, regulations, or obstacles won't change the people who don't. It created a burden only for those with good motives and intentions.

CHAPTER 9

The Ambulance Chasers

America is being overthrown by ambulance-chasing lawyers, willing to sue for the common cold if it means a dollar in their pocket. The red diaper doper babies of the 1960s (Dr. Savage has it right) have run roughshod over the American landscape, particularly in health care. What is the overall cost of these lawsuits? Who really profits? What amount of money is spent day after day due to defensive medicine? One thing is for sure; none of the money expended has or will lead to better health care.

Frivolous, uncontrolled lawsuits do not help solve problems. They only serve to line the pockets of litigators out to make a fast buck. Do bad things happen in medicine? Absolutely. Is it always someone's fault? No. In America we are sold the idea that it must always be someone's fault. Of course, no one can have individual responsibility for something that may result in a negative outcome. Individuals and ambulance-chasing attorneys have no potential impact to their life or livelihood if they file frivolous lawsuits. The cost comes to society, the system, and individual providers. Careers get ruined, insurance premiums rise to unbelievable levels, and health care loses many excellent providers who are just plain tired of the rat race imposed by the so-called do-gooders.

Malpractice or liability insurance premiums have risen to astronomical levels over the past decade. I know in my own practice that in one year the premium jumped 140 percent without ever having a claim filed. And while the practice of clinical neuropsychology has some basic risks…it's not brain surgery. Obstetricians, anesthesiologists, and surgeons must give up their firstborn in order to practice. It is commonplace for these specialties to have to pay in excess of $100,000 per year for insurance with a claim-free record. This is all before they see their first patient. It is also a major factor driving even basic health-care costs through the roof. The system cannot sustain such costs.

Defensive medicine has been undertaken in an attempt to combat litigation, but it only reinforces the idea that most professionals are not trying to do the best for their patients. There goes that trust again. Needless tests are ordered to cover one's butt. This again leads to more paperwork and more limited provider/patient interaction. As mentioned before this notion that writing more or having certain documentation provides security and better care is false. It has reached such proportions that there is software that provides "canned" documentation. Often this leads to further litigation because the software will often contradict itself. Such software is costly to develop, implement, and make useful.

One must also remember that so much of litigation is based upon the written word. As previously stated, just because it is on paper doesn't make it true. Most litigation focuses on what is written, not what is not written. Both ways lead to false assessments in many instances. Litigation does not help fix the system. Rather it focuses on a punitive approach of singling out individuals and encouraging better documentation to cover one's butt, not to be a better provider or to enhance treatment outcomes. The system has generated better writers and more people spending the bulk of their time looking over their shoulders. Your doctor is increasingly being turned into a technician rather than a clinician, exercising sound, clinical judgment. Physicians must often order tests they believe have no specific merit in a particular situation; but because there is a one in a thousand chance of something, the test gets ordered to "rule out" a disorder or ailment.

American society always has to have someone to blame. The very person that states that there must be someone at fault drives around in their VW bus with a bumper sticker that says "sh. happens" It happens every day. Unforeseen circumstances bring about negative outcomes. All sectors of life have a risk/benefit attached to them. Crossing the street may result in being hit by a car. That does not mean we shouldn't cross the street. Life doesn't come with a guarantee.

CHAPTER 10

Robbing Peter to Pay Paul

The continuing drain on our health-care system by those who don't contribute is bankrupting us as a country. The United States is the richest country on the planet but it cannot take care of the entire world's problems. Most recently we have seen an escalation in utilization by the countless numbers of illegal immigrants to the United States. These illegal immigrants may be hardworking, well-meaning individuals but typically they do not pay taxes, have insurance benefits, or have significant levels of education. Illegal immigrants do contribute to the social fabric of American society; however, they quickly bleed the system dry by extracting far more from our health care and other social systems than they put in. They obtain services through social security, Medicaid, indigent programs, emergency room access through EMTALA, anchor babies, and the overall generosity of the American public. Unfortunately, the rise in the illegal immigration population has led to the public now being played as fools. With its unprecedented speed, this problem has exponentially grown. It has grown with such vigor that the hole is so deep that it may soon be impossible to recover from it.

A skyrocketing phenomenon heading skyward even faster than health insurance premiums or costs of health care is the extraordinary burden placed on health care through illegal immigration. Current estimates suggest that between ten and twenty million illegal immigrants are currently in the United States, most of them from Mexico.

They come here illegally for a better life. Wanting a better life is a basic human desire, but at what cost? We complain daily that we cannot insure and take care of our own yet we allow the borders to remain open. Hospitals in our border towns have been closing rapidly due to our inability to pay the bills. As such we place our own legal residents at risk. They go without a place to access health care.

Illegal immigrants quickly learn the American system and how to access a myriad of social services and health care. Health care is among the most prized of the benefits from their illegal occupation of the United States. They learn that American law prohibits them from being turned away from a hospital when they present themselves in need of care. They also play on the unique altruism of America. America has always reached out but now the burden is pulling America down. We cannot continue to pay the price. In the end, we will all be left with nothing.

The cost for illegal immigrants' care does not stop with the direct provision of care. We have to communicate with them, right? So, health-care providers now need to be bilingual. There is a cost to that necessity too. Bilingual doctors, nurses, and technicians expect better pay for this added skill. Who pays for that skill? What happens if the language barrier is not conquered? It results in a lawsuit because the hospital or physician completed a procedure that was unnecessary because of faulty communication. Americans pay again.

One cannot argue that these illegal immigrants pay their fair share. Most often they do not pay taxes and if employed do not receive the benefits through their employer as part of a compensation package. This doesn't even address another sector of health care, workers' compensation. Since most of these individuals are not on the books, their employers don't pay workers' compensation insurance, so the cost gets passed on to the American taxpayer again. There is no sanction of the employer. As an employer why would you pay for such coverage when you know your employee wouldn't dream of turning you in to the authorities? You share a common bond. Employer and employee are both engaging in illegal, yet cost-saving to the employer, activities.

Numerous hospitals are seeing their resources depleted at lightning speed, so fast that the number of closures of border hospitals is becoming contagious, resulting in catastrophic failure of hospitals even in our northern states. Without change, there will be a further decline in the quality and quantity of health-care services for all. You can only rob from Peter to pay Paul for so long. Then eminent collapse comes upon us all.

The health-care crisis is not all about the strains placed upon it by utilization. It also has its looming collapse buried in the ever-growing sense of entitlement. Look at the government's recent implementation of the Medicare prescription plan. Uncle Sam has again added a benefit with a premium cost that does not pay for itself. The premium, currently about fifty to fifty-five dollars a month, gives Medicare recipients access to a medicine cabinet full of medicine. This population has the highest utilization rate. As we get older, we are more likely to need health care and therefore medicine. We didn't hear anything from the AARP contingency about eliminating another benefit to help offset cost. All we heard is that our seniors deserve a prescription benefit and with the help of AARP, the pharmaceutical lobby, and others in a position of potential political or economic gain, they got it.

The Medicare and Medicaid systems even before the implementation of the new prescription plan were a disaster. Uncle Sam has no business in the health-care field. Like almost everything else, it has screwed the system up beyond repair. Do you ever wonder what people did prior to the start of LBJ's Great Society? Didn't people get and pay for health care? Uncle Sam is not a health-care provider or an efficient payer source. The government engaging in oversight can be a good thing in setting guidelines, but it should not dictate what can and cannot be done in health care. Uncle Sam did not attend medical school.

CHAPTER 11

Oh, Doc, My Back's Killing Me

That phrase is the battle cry of the workers' compensation and social security disability patient. They become injured on the job or in some other situation and quickly become indoctrinated into "the system." They are told by workers' compensation attorneys or social security attorneys not to push too hard for recovery. After all, the quicker you get well, the less benefits that are available at the end of the rainbow. There are no incentives to remain independent. Funny thing is, however, once a settlement in the worker compensation case or social security case occurs, a magical cure for the ailment seems to surface. These people then become the double dippers. They receive benefits from an insurance company or social security while getting jobs that pay under the table. Yes, you and your neighbor get the short stick again. Social security gets closer to bankruptcy, and costs to employers for workers' compensation insurance rise, which is in turn passed on to the consumer in the way of the higher cost of goods.

Many will say I don't know what I am talking about. Rubbish. I have seen it every day in my practice. Granted not all those applying for Social Security Disability Insurance or those with workers' compensation injuries are users but the numbers are significant. In my own practice, I have had a number of Social Security attorneys refer patients for an evaluation for either mental health or neurological, particularly postconcussion, syndromes in order to get Social

Security benefits. Most of the attorneys stopped referring when in the evaluation of their clients I would ask, "How did you get to my office?"

They would usually reply, "I drove myself in a car." I would then have to tell them that they didn't qualify for Social Security benefits because they could hold competitive employment as a driver, courier, etc. The regulations state any job, not one that you would necessarily like. We aren't entitled to the "perfect job or career."

Workers' compensation insurance companies also spend millions upon millions of dollars in fraud detection of "injured workers" who scam the system. They supposedly have a bad back from the work injury, yet they are caught on film lifting landscape boulders to make the new retaining wall at their house paid for from disability payments provided by the insurance carrier/employer.

Workers' compensation attorneys also get huge sums of money for work that should not even be necessary. The workers' compensation system in most states is pretty straightforward once the employer has admitted liability. So why an attorney if the system is in place? It would seem a better fix is tightening up the enforcement of workers' compensation laws, a one-time fix, rather than ongoing litigation with no fix and higher costs. Come on, people. We are smart. The fix can't be just political. It must be win-win for everyone.

The personal injury forum suffers from many of the same issues. It is adversarial and the system wants to blame someone and subsequently make them pay. In many jurisdictions, the "injured "party" has nothing to lose. They engage an attorney who often becomes more of a negotiator in settling. The other party, often the insurance company, must make a business decision often that frequently comes down to dollars and cents. They must calculate the cost to litigate, time, experts, etc. They often settle because it is cheaper to do so. The insurance company in turn recoups much of the money via rising premiums. The cost is passed on to the consumer.

CHAPTER 12

Diagnose the Problem
Now What's the Cure?

In the first half of this surgical strike on health care, we have engaged in exploratory surgery. We have opened up the system and looked at its symptoms and even found cancer in some areas. In this next procedure, we will embark on the use of mainstream techniques, surgical techniques of cutting out the bad, radiating the cancer, and bandaging the wounds where possible to encourage proper healing. We know from our exploration that the system is irrevocably broken and can no longer be treated with a Band-Aid and a cold compress. We must simultaneously look at all the areas of pathology and work to implement a system that cuts out the cancer but allows the system to be reborn. Treatment must be multifaceted and no system can be left untreated, for if not treated, the pathology will return if only in another form.

The identified symptoms have been found to be the insurance industry, government, consumers/patients, big business, bureaucracy, providers, greed, politics, mistrust, litigation, and entitlement. All these symptoms must be addressed with a vengeance. Failure to do so will result in the cancer of health care eating a part the fabric of American society from the inside out. We are approaching a point of terminal care if a cure is not undertaken quickly.

What is the cure for American health care? I will now attempt to expound on treatments and interventions aimed at treating the etiology of the crisis in American health care. Such treatment will be much like treating a cancer. It must be radical in some respects but it has gone on much too long. We can no longer pretend the disease is not there. It is quickly moving from an insidious ailment to Americans and is now raving the system and will not survive without radical, purposeful, steadfast intervention.

All Americans Must Be a Part of the System and Treatment

First, Americans must return to their propensity for altruism. We are all in this boat together. American society must come together for the greater whole. Factions cannot say, for whatever reason, I will not participate. People can give a multitude of reasons why they should not be included; however, sooner or later, we all must access the health-care system and therefore a sharing of health care responsibility in a basic tenet of our society and culture.

Immediately many individuals will indicate, "I don't need coverage. I am young and healthy." In general, they are correct. Common sense as well as statistics would indicate that fact. Unfortunately, life does not come with a crystal ball. We are unable to unequivocally predict our health-care needs and future. Even when chances of the need to access and have the necessary medical treatment are small, the percentage is still there. Even if the chances are ninety-nine to one, someone must be the 1 percent. When it is ourselves, we don't want to wish you had had the forethought to plan.

A person quickly responds that they are being forced to be included and pay for the necessary insurance. While currently against the US Constitution, an individual cannot be forced to purchase any product, in this case health insurance; revisions must be made. The reasoning for such is on various fronts.

In practicality, each individual in the United States receives health care to a greater or lesser extent. They, in large part, do not go without. That is a huge credit to the American people. Unlike many of the world's countries, we do not turn the sick person out into the streets because they have an inability to pay. Up to now we have dealt with this through voluntary participation in health insurance. Whatever the reasons for nonparticipation, we, as a free society, have allowed people to make the choice. It may be because they don't think they need it, I can't afford it, and so on.

What happens when people without a means of reimbursing the system access health care? Sure, the system attempts to recoup the expenditures for their care; but as the old saying goes, "You can't get blood out of a turnip." Then what happens? The individual has a cost for the care but can't pay for it. Well, most often the cost is then shifted to those in the system that do have the means and insurance. The cost of procedures, treatments, and intervention is placed upon them. It is much like what was mentioned earlier. They are essentially shoplifters at your local Walmart. They get an item but don't have to pay for it. Walmart attempts to recoup the cost from the individual if caught. Most often they cannot provide restitution. They are then shunned by many parts of society. What is Walmart forced to do to the shoplifter…the cost of all other items in the store are raised to offset the losses of the shoplifter, and then the paying customer pays the price. Health-care reimbursement for nonpayment is no different.

Financial ruin is also a common occurrence when individuals cannot pay for their health care. This is even true when the individual does have health insurance—just not enough of it or a policy that does not cover the medical intervention supplied. This results in bankruptcy, credit impairment, garnishing of wages, and even having to choose between treatment and/or medicine and their ability to supply food and shelter to themselves and family members.

One of the biggest reasons all individuals must be part of the system is the result of basic statistics. Insurance companies try to cherry-pick their insured. They cherry-pick those individuals who they perceive as the lowest risk and therefore have the least number of claims and cost. In general, they want young healthy individuals with minimal or no medical problems. They certainly do not prefer older people because the older we get, the more likely we are to need medical intervention and subsequent cost. Insurance companies also want to exclude preexisting conditions as those conditions are a known infringement on profits. Insurance companies must insure all *preexisting* diagnoses. There must also be *no* lifetime cap on benefits. Remember, we are all in this boat together and must row as such.

By having all people insured, the "sample" is then totally random and will result in the statistical bell-shaped curve. In other words, by not including or excluding people, a true cross section is derived. This includes all individuals with any type of preexisting condition. Participation by everyone will help assure that the population is not favorably or unfavorably looked upon by others. Certain parameters are no longer parceled out to the advantage of the insurance carriers' profits. Remembering that insurance is *shared risk*, all insured people now equally share in that risk. Not having the crystal ball, all people are equally covered. Of course, we all hope for the best but must plan for the worst. That is what insurance is all about.

Nonprofit

The current system has both for-profit and nonprofit insurance carriers and institutions such as hospitals. The argument is often cited by individuals that through competition and capitalism innovation will prosper and cost will be lower. Unfortunately, in such a system, it is assumed that the system is driven by typical capitalistic principles of the free market. One of those principles is that capitalism operates under free choice. Individuals do or do not purchase goods and services based on need, want, monetary means, and the like. It is voluntary.

Health care and its subsequent reimbursement are almost never voluntary except when you must see your plastic surgeon to assure yourself you will be young forever. Health care is essentially a forced choice. No one says to their friend, "I think I will go see my physician on Tuesday. I have nothing else to do." People go and get medical treatment because they need it. Even then they don't and can't say they want to save money. When a person shops for a refrigerator, they typically have a budget but yet have certain features that they would like to have. It might be the stainless steel. That icemaker in the door. They budget $1,500. They arrive at the appliance store only to find the refrigerator they want is $2,000. Being well above their budget, they decide they can only afford the regular black one with the icemaker inside. It is the $1,500. They do so because the choice is voluntary and meets their budget. This is not true of medical treatment. You cannot go into your surgeon and say, "Hey, Doc, I want to save $500, so skip the sutures." It is forced upon us, nonvoluntary, and most likely an all-or-nothing proposition.

A for-profit model also takes advantage of an individual's misfortune and makes a profit from something inherently needed by all. It is like charging for the air we breathe. We really don't have a choice and become captive. An individual that purchases shares in an insurance company or for-profit hospital chain expects to make a dividend. They don't buy it to break even. The company's motive is always making the most profit for the company. As such, they might deny service and make it more difficult to access service via limited providers, hospitals., etc. They attempt to place as many obstacles in the way as they can. For-profit hospitals may become more worried about wallpaper than stellar care. Anything that may result in profit. Once again profits largely go into the pockets of shareholders and not optimal care, research, staff hiring, and ratios.

Of course, one can easily say nonprofits can be manipulated to essentially be a for-profit structure. Paper losses are tied up in astronomical salaries of administrators, CEOs, board members, nicer buildings, and all the other trappings. That is not to say payment for talented people should not happen or buildings should be nothing more than shells. There must be a reasonable medium and objective oversight of such must be in place. Nonprofit status and its manipulation must also be tightened up and return to what we all think of as nonprofit. There must be enough money coming in the front door to pay for the expenses going out the back door. Nonprofit status is also much more appropriate for a system we all must contribute to because of necessity and one we will all access sooner or later.

One Plan

Much like necessary inclusion in participation to insurance, there should only be one plan of coverage. As it stands now, there is a myriad of plans, all with different coverages and different costs—indemnity plans, HMOs, PPOs, capitation, Medicare, Medicaid, indigent, Veterans Administration, workers' compensation, and personal injury. Each has its own coverage, cost, infrastructure, reimbursement, and bureaucracy. Each has its own administration, rules, regulations, pluses, and minuses. Each of these things come with a cost.

While there are literally hundreds of insurance plans across the country, all with different coverage, different qualifications, and different costs, their intent is to cover but one type of thing…the human body. While there are different sexes, ethnicity, genetic and pregenetic traits, diseases, and injuries, the goal is to cover the medical-related cost of the human body. People are unable even with the advancement of science and medicine to achieve the predictability inherent in humans. We cannot see the medical needs of an individual into the future. We might know some probabilities but not assurances. By only having these probabilities, what plan do I pick? What if I pick the wrong plan and the medical intervention I need is not covered? With our current system, this scenario happens every day. If you choose the wrong plan and one aspect is not covered, it is just like having no insurance at all. Therefore, the cost is again shifted to others via charity, government, and you as the taxpayer. There is no way to predict with certainty the needs of a specific individual.

How is such a dilemma fixed? One plan. The question only becomes what plan with what coverage? Eighty-twenty plan, ninety-ten, PPO, HMO? Maybe 100 percent? What diagnoses? What procedures? These are all questions that must be answered but society must do it as a whole. The plan must then be universal; otherwise, cost is eventually shifted.

Having multiple plans would certainly work in a typical capitalistic environment; but as discussed earlier, this is not a typical environment that is voluntary. The incorporation of one plan results in the need for much less administration on the part of insurance companies, as well as providers. Employees of the insurance companies no longer have to know countless plan coverages. Providers can have much less in the way of front office people navigating the red tape and bureaucracy. All the trappings of marketing multiple products also are eliminated, thereby reducing plan administration cost.

The simplicity for the consumer also becomes evident. One plan provides for more straightforward understanding of coverage—less hassle for what is or is not covered. Having only one plan, of which everyone is included, makes the randomness more authentic and based on equal probability inherent in the bell-shaped curve.

Another potential variable within the single plan would be equality of premiums. No matter what age, sex, ethnicity, etc., the premium is always the same. Probability would suggest, for example, that younger people get sick less than older people and need less medical care. In general, that is true. If the odds are with you, you need less care and therefore would have less cost. You ask then, "Shouldn't a young person pay less?" We must remember: insurance is a *shared risk*. We must be willing to share equally throughout life since it is impossible to predict the future, and after all we are insuring the future.

Multiple Insurance Carriers

Multiple insurance carriers would assure continuity. They would be much like the nonprofit health insurance companies evident prior to the mid-1980s. The availability of multiple companies would be akin to the various charities—Goodwill, Salvation Army, UNICEF, and so forth. Since there would not be competition, as such the number of insurance carriers would significantly decrease. One thing is quite clear. The government should not be in the business of insurance company. Like almost all government-run programs, it would be coupled with bureaucracy, redundancy, corruption, and frequently incompetence. There would be a place for the government to be in the position of oversight.

Simple Reimbursement System

Having been in direct health care for almost thirty years, I have seen and experienced the nightmares associated with health-care reimbursement. I have seen where a physician practice has to have more people in the front office than in the back. This is necessary to obtain the necessary paperwork, authorization, preauthorization, calling insurance companies to verify coverage, in network, out of network, determining what the coverage will be, co-pays, deductibles, and on and on. Hospitals are fraught with much of the same thing. Additionally, coders search charts for diagnosis to maximize payment.

The insurance companies also have numerous people to provide authorization, case management, utilization, customer service to provide verification of coverage, and many more. Layers upon layers. Each layer costing health-care dollars, thereby increasing the cost of health care to the end user, the consumer (patient).

Of course, all positions would not be eliminated; however, the streamlining of both sides of the equation would lead to a much simpler, quicker, more efficient system. On top of that technology is rapidly evolving which could further simplify the reimbursement process. Even the submission of a claim is daunting. Approximately 10 percent of all health-care costs are associated with collection of that dollar. That is ten cents to collect every dollar. Remarkable. How can it be that companies like Visa, Mastercard, and American Express can have a much more streamlined system and on average only charge the merchant 3 percent? Claims have become much more universal, yet insurance companies and providers still utilize clearinghouses to make claims more universal. That middleman does not do it for free! Another unnecessary cost inherent in the system.

Incentives for Providers and Institutions

Within the concept of universal health care, government-based health care, and socialized medicine is the idea of mediocrity. Even in our current system, some of those pitfalls exist. If I am a physician and, in this model, I make the same monetarily as a colleague but I work twice as hard and I am twice as good, why strive to excel? Many do not. It strips away incentives of all kinds. It curtails innovation, intelligence, and pride of the individual. Institutions as a whole are saddled with similar problems. If they are all put on the same level, why be the best? The best should be rewarded. There is a difference between the Mayo Clinic and Acme Medical. As such they should be rewarded and commended. Much better, quantifiable measures need to be instilled. These measures and expectations must be universal and determined objectively and not filled with fluff. This might include lower death rates, shorter lengths of stay with decreased complications, lower rates of hospital-borne infections, etc.

Incentives might occur to institutions via higher rates of reimbursement, more grants, higher objective ratings, and so forth. Individual practitioners might have other incentives. If they are superior, they should be compensated as such. As the system now stands, you could be the best heart surgeon in the world or the worst and reimbursement from insurance company A is essentially the same. It is even more evident when an internist gets reimbursement from an insurance company set on a fee schedule. For better or worse. Hence, to accommodate this fact, internists are forced to see more and more patients to increase compensation. It results in essentially drive-by doctors' visits. You are not compensated by knowledge, skill, or experience.

The fee schedule for a certain procedure through a certain insurance company is determined; and no matter your length of experience, skill, or knowledge, you are compensated the same. Additionally, most insurance companies do not allow any billing of the patient beyond their co-pay or deductible.

One possible way to compensate and provide a practitioner with incentive might be via a predetermined amount that the insurance company proves for a service. Whether you are good or bad, you receive the same. Then if the practitioner believes he/she is "worth," it then may charge more than the reimbursement rate provided by the insurance company. The practitioner is then able to bill the patient for the difference. The control and choice is thereby up to the patient. Like any service, they will be willing to pay for it. If the practitioner has a higher rate, they would only establish it if they can get it. Basic supply and demand as well as fair compensation for being the best.

Government Removal from Health-Care Reimbursement

The largest "health insurance company" in the United States is the government, particularly the Medicare program. It also sponsors the Medicaid programs, Veterans Administration, and various smaller programs. The common denominator in each is bureaucracy, fraud, abuse, poor care, depleted levels of reimbursement, and insolvency. Each of these programs has layers and layers of bureaucracy. There are so many regulations of what you can and can't do, how to do this or that, and crippled implementation of health care itself. With these layers and layers of bureaucracy, there is fraud well beyond any private sector company. This is compounded by programs that are ever-expanding. Benefits become more and more without a means of paying for them. Each benefit may be worthwhile but with that comes cost. Legislation is passed and politicians typically have enhanced allegiance from their contingents. Reelection becomes more ensured while the cost is on the back of taxpayers. Politicians allow lobbying groups like insurance companies and pharmaceutical companies to fill their war chest for that next election and for that golden parachute.

Programs like the Veterans Administration are filled with many of the same problems. They must even have the added burden of having hospitals, physicians, and providers directly working within the system. They are overwhelmed, shorthanded, and frequently working with less-than-optimal resources.

All these programs should be returned to the private sector. It would simplify the overall system through one plan. Furthermore, since everyone is included in the system, there would no longer be a population skewing such as the elderly in the Medicare program, indigent in the Medicaid program, or veterans in the Veterans Administration. The providers and facilities would no longer be needed in the Veterans Administration as it would be absorbed into the private sector. As such the government would save administration cost, personnel cost, and facility cost.

Similar savings would be achieved when all these other programs are to the private sector. Of course, programs such as Medicare would need to be transitioned back to the private sector as it has been so entrenched in the government and as an entitlement program. A complete elimination or overnight replacement would most probably be overwhelming to health care and the overall US economy. The country did not find itself in this dilemma overnight. It was gradual and oftentimes insidious. More often than not, the changes, additions, or deletions were largely politically motivated. The country can no longer kick the can down the road. The lack of addressing this aspect of the government is increasingly eating the very fabric of America from the inside out. There must be a fundamental change in the public's belief that it is the role of the government to play the role of caretaker and in its place have it replaced with individual responsibility.

Government Oversight

As mentioned above, the government acting as the insurance company on the federal or state level is fraught with countless pitfalls. The few attempts at intervening to fix these pitfalls have been putting our finger in the dam while water is gushing over the spillway. Piecemeal intervention does not work. It begins with the idea that it is the government's job to provide health care. A theory riddled in fallacy. Aggressive movement must be undertaken to correct this fallacy. Simultaneously, the government should play the irreplaceable role of oversight. This is necessary to provide the requisite provisions to have checks and balances. This is invaluable to assure that all citizens have this function fulfilled when essentially having a public-private partnership.

While insurance companies would be in the private sector and that all citizens would partake in such a health-care revision, there still may be unforeseen aspects of administration, implementation, and ongoing provision of it. The analogy that might be employed here is that of the Federal Aviation Administration (FAA). While the FAA does not provide airlines and other airline functions, it is responsible for the oversight and regulation of the airline industry. It has established regulations, policies, and procedures for the industry to have and follow. It is with such a system that countless functions of the industry are provided. One of the overriding aspects of their oversight is the safety of the American public. This oversight would need to be needed in much the same way. In eliminating federal and state programs, the government can allow the private sector to manage health care in a much more systematic, less bureaucratic way.

Universal System

As previously addressed, there are multiple systems currently in the overall health-care system. This is on both clinical and financial levels. Many of their threads have commonality but operate redundantly and frequently inadequately. There are systems such as Medicare, Medicaid, Veterans Administration, workers' compensation, personal injury, and public and private sectors. Federal, state, and even local government play roles as well.

Payment and clinical tenets are quite frequently fighting against one another. They quite often run parallel parameters which leads to a lack of cooperation and unnecessary redundancy in the overall system. While the government should not remain a payer, and certainly should not become a single payer, the oversight as mentioned earlier can go far to eliminating the lack of cooperation and redundancy on both clinical and financial levels.

Examples of such a collapse can be found in the collapsing of the Veterans Administration. Such a consolidation can occur both clinically and financially. Clinically, it is inefficient to have both facilities and health-care staff solely within the VA system. Why do the VA and our government need separate clinics, hospitals, and other points of entry? The VA can handle placing all its patients into the private system—that system having its own facilities. As a result, the VA, and therefore our government, saves hundreds of millions of dollars annually. The same is true with the providers. Why are separate doctors, nurses, and so on needed? Clinically, all those needs can be meet in the single model proposed. Once again, vast amounts of money are saved by the government/taxpayer; and layers upon layers of red tape are eliminated, thus saving money again.

Certainly, the veterans and personnel of our country deserve outstanding health care from the best the country has to offer. They should not be quarantined to a small fraction of the health-care system. After all, these men and women risked their lives to defend our freedom and assure we continue to make the American way of life envied by the world.

How would this be paid for? Just as in the private sector, employers and even individuals would have a premium paid each month to cover their military-related care. The stipend would be paid directly to the insurance company of the veterans' choice just as would be seen in the private arena. Oversight could be afforded as well vis-à-vis what the government outlined previously. VA benefits, if you will, would be overseen by an arm of this agency.

The workers' compensation system would work in much the same fashion. While that system does not have facilities to construct and maintain, many providers practice almost exclusively within the workers' compensation system. That system tends to have very adversarial aspects and as such prolongs treatment in many cases and promotes secondary gain.

Employers currently pay premiums to a separate, workers' compensation-only insurance company. The collapsing of health-care aspects of workers' compensation through one single type of health insurance would go a long way to minimize redundancy and aspects of secondary gain, lessen the adversarial roles currently in the system, and streamline payment of the care. In the single care model, employers would be directing premium dollars to the various private sector insurance companies.

Personal injury insurance for other types of injuries is presently, usually accessed through automobile insurance claims, business liability insurance, etc. It, too, can amount to adversarial relationships and impediments in the provision of care, thereby prolonging the process. Delay in the acceptance of liability is seen often. Under the single care model, care is no longer delayed or tied up in the liability question. Care is provided while the question of liability is sorted out among the interested parties. Efficiency is the key to treatment and therefore cost.

The Medicare system, government-run and sanctioned, is for individuals sixty-five and older, as well as the disabled who qualify. It is a program initiated and mandated by the federal government. It is a system that has countless problems inherent to most governmental programs—fraud, abuse, overuse, and bureaucratic inefficiency. It has also become a political pawn used by politicians as a carrot to attract the votes of retirees and the older generation. This is seen via the constant expansion of benefits without the necessary increase in personal revenue contribution. It is through and through an entitlement program.

The Medicare system is failing and for many years it has not been sustaining itself. Benefits are expanded and people are living longer, thereby needing to access care for a longer period of time. It is also the program that insures the ever-expanding elderly population so their amount of insured accessing health care at any given time is growing. By definition the older we get, the more individuals are likely to need health care. Due to the many reasons delineated above, this program needs replacement. It is unlikely that this replacement will come overnight for both practical and political reasons. To address this problem and to move toward a single care model, strategic steps in a finite manner must be implemented. For a whole host of reasons, benefits cannot be stripped away in order to have solvency. Hence, the plan of attack must be incremental.

Therefore, the program must be rolled back and shifted to the private insurance sector in steps. For example, the prescription benefit available to recipients might be moved into the private sector. All other benefits would initially remain with the Medicare program. The prescription benefit would then be transferred to private insurance carriers like other health care will be. The associated benefits and associated premiums and cost paid by the recipients and government would then be directed to the private sector. This would begin to get the government out of the health insurance business, reduce cost based upon greater *shared risk*, and eliminate countless governmental agencies tasked with administration of this runaway train and entitlement.

Each segment of the Medicare program would be systematically taken over by the private insurance companies. This approach might initially include all Medicare B (most outpatient services) which are currently paid for, and is voluntary to the beneficiary, and subsided by additional government dollars.

Eventually, Medicare A benefits (mostly inpatient services) would be transferred to the private sector. This is the portion of Medicare that is a mandatory deduction from payroll. Again, it is a portion of the program which is not self-sustaining. It may be necessary to gradually phase out this aspect of the program. One methodology may be the gradual transfer of these benefits on a percentage basis. For example, initially the government continues to pay 70 percent of these services, while 30 percent is directed with the appropriate percentage of premium dollars (e.g., payroll deduction) absorbed by the private sector.

To a certain extent, this type of methodology would be similar to the currently available Medicare-managed care plans. These are the programs set up by private insurance companies to manage Medicare benefits while receiving a stipend from the government when an individual assigns their benefits to them.

Eventually through this systematic plan, the payroll deduction would be eliminated, and the money saved by the individual would then be directed through their choice of insurance companies. It increases the individual control and has the government limit its role in health care. It should also be added that the progressive inclusion of the Medicare population to the overall population of insured will become increasingly balanced resulting in more of a true bell-shaped curve and equal distribution of risk and cost. In other words, the sickest portion of the population, elderly, will now include the healthiest portion of the population, children. Cost is then spread out along the entire spectrum and not skewed to include only a segment of the entire universe of lives that need to be insured.

The Medicaid and other programs are government sponsored and should be handled in a similar way. Since Medicaid and similar programs usually focus on the lowest strata of the socioeconomic ladder, it is the government/taxpayer that foots the bill. Again, these programs have become obsolete, burdensome, and increasingly costly. Including these recipients in the collective population of all insured will further increase their having access to all health care while eliminating the government as a quasi-insurance company. Once again, the risks are mutually shared.

Elimination of all Medical and Pharmaceutical Advertisement

Some research suggests that the United States may consume as much as 75 percent of the world's pharmaceuticals yet is only 5 percent of the world population. Hospitals are increasingly advertising one service or another. Medical equipment companies do much the same. If you speak with these industries, you will most frequently hear that the public has the right to know and be educated. Unfortunately, the education only comes in the form of marketing to sell their product. Their Madison Avenue cohorts synthesize commercials, print ads, and radio spots only to sell products. The consumer is told that they need this drug to eliminate, minimize, or enhance their lives. This approach neglects to indicate all the other possible interventions to address the problem. That may be another medication, physical therapy, ultrasound, surgery, and so forth. They hock their product like it is the best thing since sliced bread, all the while minimizing to the greatest extent possible. The American consumer becomes convinced that the product is a must-have to address the real or even perceived medical calamity. It reinforces the Western philosophy, especially the American one, that there is a pill for everything.

The prevalence of pharmaceuticals has proliferated ever since advertisement came into being in the mid-1980s. Data suggests that the pharmaceutical industry spends approximately 10 percent of the total expenditure for pharmaceuticals each year. That expenditure is currently 325 billion dollars. Previously, pharmaceuticals were presented to the patient through their physician or health-care provider. It was their job, and ethical obligation, to present *all* the treatment alternatives available to that patient. Hence, the decision of what intervention, if any, was between the doctor and the patient.

It was only then that true education occurred and the best treatment employed. At present, the patient/consumer sees a commercial, hears an advertisement, or reads in a magazine that medicine X is the answer. The patient then goes to their doctor and insists that the medicine they saw is the answer. Even when the physician informs the patient that it may not be the best course, increasing pressure to prescribe the medication ensues. When the physician puts down their foot, he/she sometimes risks the loss of a patient because they have been told that this is the answer. These many times lead to doctor shopping until the patient hears and subsequently gets what they want.

Health-care facilities such as hospitals, clinics, MRIs, colonoscopies, and so forth have led to inappropriate use and overutilization. Radio spots will say, "You better go out and get your heart scan right away or you may be a heart attack waiting to happen." They will even add that it is no problem because your insurance will pay for it. The consumer reacts, "Great." They feel it is no skin off their back.

Digressing for a moment but indicative of a clear example is a television ad produced for *Stryker* hip prosthesis some time ago. It featured Arnold Palmer, the great golfer, indicating his terrific experience when a *Stryker* was used in his hip replacement. It made me chuckle thinking that a person who is in need must in part to their orthopedic surgeon before surgery that, "Hey, Doc. Make sure you use *Stryker* hip prosthesis. Don't go using that *Ace Hardware* stuff!" It is comical because the patient obviously would not know one hip prosthesis from another and which one might be best.

The elimination of all advertisement would enhance health care and curtail unnecessary intervention and therefore cost. Providers would no longer have to navigate and undo the promises of the industry's pitchmen.

Fee Disclosure

Rarely are fees and cost discussed with the patient. The patient is frequently told, "No problem, your insurance will cover it." Furthermore, the patient, especially on an inpatient hospital stay, is already apprehensive, vulnerable, and even scared. That often seems to be an invitation of carte blanche by the hospital. The patient is never informed that that plastic disposable urinal is fifty dollars. They are easily exploited.

Routinely, payment of services is made directly to the provider, and the patient may never see a bill until an explanation of benefits (EOB) eventually arrives. Frequently, the EOB arrives with surprise, surprise. Many things were not covered by insurance and your bill is...all too often the bill is beyond the means of the patient and creates hardship, and even sometimes it results in bankruptcy. It ruins lives.

In the old days, so to speak payment was made to the patient not directly to the provider. It may seem like an unnecessary step and inconvenient; however, when this occurred and the patient saw the bill directly, it had great psychological meaning. The patient recognized that high costs may be involved, billing may be incorrect, and there is a connection with all aspects of health care and the personal responsibilities accompanying it.

Bottom line, fees should be disclosed. You never just let your plumber or electrician charge whatever they want. You generally know what is coming. Health care should be no different.

Independence of Providers and Institutions

In recent years there has been a gradual blending of provider practices and hospitals. There are various reasons for such, ranging from physicians wanting to be clinicians and not business people, consolidation of overhead cost, increasing direct referrals from physician offices to hospitals, increased control by hospitals of their providers, and monetary increases via owning various practices. Generally, this would seem to be a good idea, but in practicality it is accompanied by various problems.

Under the previous model, physicians and hospitals were totally independent from one another. Physicians obtained staff privileges at the hospital(s) where they practiced. Hospitals established criteria to obtain those privileges. Each was independent from one another. They were not financially or clinically together. Each entity was responsible for their domain. That model has been changing. Hospitals are now owning practices, physicians are employed directly by hospitals, and physicians have lost much of their independent clinical judgment.

First and foremost, when the entities were totally separate, the physician's clinical judgment was independent. They prescribed the tests, treatment, lengths of stay, etc. They were independent in their judgment as to what patients needed. This began to change with the bleeding of one entity with another. One now had a vested interest in the other. For example, if a physician believes a patient needs more time in the hospital, a certain test, etc., there may be implicit or explicit direction from administration. Often it is related to business or financial aspects of a case. The independence gets lost. Pressure may come to decrease or increase service in some way. Clinical judgment may be impeded consciously or unconsciously. Separateness seems to have been better from a health-care perspective. Also, increased medical management leads to lower cost overall.

The overlap between providers and institutions has also seen the advent of all providers having services that were previously independent. Such a case is in the case of an OB-GYN physician that now has ultrasound equipment directly in their office. They may have a tendency, either implicitly or explicitly, to order that test even when it is clinically questionable. They convince the patient and sometimes themselves that it is more "convenient" within the confines of their office. In actuality it may be a profit center for the practice or they just bought new equipment they want to pay for via these tests.

The same can be said of laboratory tests. Previously, the physician wrote a prescription and sent you off to get your blood drawn at the hospital. Now the physician may have certain laboratory tests available directly in their office.

Physicians also may own a freestanding MRI and advertise to have your heart scan done as a preventative measure. While many times the test may be indicated, other times this may not be the case, clouded by financial incentive.

Universal Credentialing

Many steps have been taken to provide a more straightforward process of credentialing professionals. This may include insurance companies, hospitals, nursing homes, and more. Each entity has its own format, forms, and way of credentialing. Common criteria and process must be adopted. At present, there can be different provider numbers, different obstacles, etc. Such differences result in time, confusion, redundancy, and as a result money spent which could be better spent on direct care.

Credentialing has even included various insurance panels that credential providers as being in network or out of network. Insurance companies will often deny joining a panel indicating it is "closed." One would think the insurance company would want to have as many providers that are qualified on their panel so that choice is increased with their insured. This is often not the case. Insurance companies are able to indirectly have some level of control over providers.

Under the one plan system, panels would be eliminated. If an individual meets the universal criteria established, they are then able to accept that insurance. The patient regains control and choice.

Elimination of Preauthorization

Many insurance plans now have preauthorization before procedures, tests, surgery, etc. can be undertaken. They often justify this gatekeeper function as necessary to increase clinical management. More often than not, it is to delay or deny the service as a money-saving endeavor. They frequently make such decisions without ever meeting or assessing the patient, or the decision is made through insurance personnel that have much less training than the person treating the patient. This can result in an adversarial relationship with your own insurance company. One must remember that the goal of the insurance company is to generate revenue in some way and not to make sure the patient receives all they need.

The process of preauthorization quite frequently takes time, energy, telephone calls, written correspondence, and so on. The provider spends the time and energy without any compensation. As such this keeps them from helping others. The insurance company must also hire and process these requests. A big circle can get created with the patient stuck in the middle. It comes down to "time is money." This is true for both sides of the equation.

Under the idea of one plan, it would explicitly dictate what is and is not covered and the reimbursement associated with that medical intervention. Clinical direction is then left up to the clinician in conjunction with the patient.

Insurance and Person are Inseparable

To enhance parsimony and to promote control by the patient, insurance must be able to follow the patient. Having a single plan also helps. Insurance companies will be chosen based mostly on their service. It will not be chosen by employer, slick marketing campaigns, or plans that are so filled with exceptions and fine print that the advantage goes to the patient.

In addition to the insurance and person being inseparable, the purchase must be able with no curtailing by laws forbidding a company not being to write across state lines. This is especially true with the current progression of technology. Simplicity must reign.

Revision of HIPPA and ADA guidelines

Both the HIPPA and the ADA were well intentioned but in practice have become cumbersome and costly. As such a much-needed cost-benefit analysis must be undertaken and a return to common sense. I have even seen that ongoing confusion resulting in fear of noncompliance, fines, and lack of communication. Many indirect costs are incurred through these acts. For example, a parking lot at your local strip mall must have a certain ratio of handicap parking slots. This is even the case when the volume does not suggest the need for so many spots. Hence, land is not allowed to serve another purpose, costing owners money for nonuse. Retrofitting of buildings for accessibility results in undue financial outlay, sometimes even causing a business not to be able to operate. All should be treated equally but the handicapped should not incur a distinct advantage because of the acts.

Direct health care must also error on the side of individual well-being. I discussed earlier something as simple as communication can result in care issues due to the need for privacy. It can even rise to the level of being life-threatening. Practicality and common sense must supersede things that are "only by the book."

Reasonable Consolidation of Facilities

The infrastructure of brick-and-mortar facilities has reached new heights—countless minor emergency room facilities, urgent care centers, freestanding surgery centers, and MRIs. Some of these facilities are affiliated with hospitals, while others stand on their own. We see the facilities cropping up to act as a feeder system to hospitals' convenience and even centers primarily aimed at profit. The construction and maintenance cost money and many are not needed. They have led to fragmentation in the delivery system and propagated needless cost and utilization. An examination of where such facilities are must be undertaken and the subsequent elimination of many in urban areas. Instead, viability in rural areas where access to resources can be difficult should be undertaken.

Tort Reform

The United States is the most litigious society in the world. Essentially you can sue for anything.

Certainly, one must be able to correct the wrongs thrust upon the citizens. Unfortunately, the growing lack of common sense, lack of personal responsibility, and trial lawyers whose motivation is often driven by the cash cow has led to defensive medicine, outrageous malpractice, insurance premiums, frivolous lawsuits, and increases in the adversarial posture of Americans.

Hospitals and doctors alike find the need to order tests, procedures, and treatments in order to cover their butts. Clinically they may not be inclined to do many things but have become forced to just to avoid any chance at litigation. This results in untold amount of money being spent to reduce any such possibility. As such, the cost is passed on to the payers of health care. It is embedded in the cost of providing care. Expenditures that often should not be there. In turn, this has resulted in an escalation in malpractice and liability insurance. It has risen to the level that physicians must give up their practice because the cost of insurance has become too high. Malpractice insurance carriers have been caused to no longer insure institutions due to the volume of lawsuits.

Attorneys will often bring lawsuits on behalf of individuals that have more than questionable parameters. They are willing to "take the chance" since most often they have no skin in the game and can only be the recipient of positive outcomes. Often, attorneys do the math as do individuals and businesses that find out that it is cheaper to settle than to litigate. These expenditures are then passed on to the end user, often the patient.

Solutions must be realized whereby everyone has skin in the game and all parties must have a consequence. If the party believes they were wronged, they should certainly stand up for that cause. At the same time, they should not be able to bring action just because an accident or unfortunate event occurs. Sometimes bad things just happen.

Illegal Immigration and the Quest of American Health Care to Support the World

A growing problem in the United States is the rampant growth of illegal immigration and its impact on American culture and the health-care system. This problem has largely been evident in the larger cities and throughout the country. It has hit border towns on the southern border. For example, Mexican expectant women have crossed the border in order to give birth to an anchor baby. It gives citizenship to these children and many of the social safety nets available. In doing so the utilization of hospitals in towns like San Diego. The lack of insurance and financial resources have left hospitals holding the bag for hundreds of thousands of dollars in unpaid care. It is also seen in cities where illegal immigrants who work at minimum wage jobs or under-the-table positions access health care via emergency rooms without resources to pay for the services. The treatment in emergency rooms is one of the most expensive venues to obtain care in. Once again hospitals lose the revenue and it has to be absorbed by others. The system is being overrun. This, in turn, eventually causes the closing of hospitals or the severe curtailment of services in order to survive. The only reasonable intervention is the severe and decisive stoppage of illegal immigration. Even those altruistic individuals who want to say it is a human right have to admit the relentless provision of care without payment cannot be sustained. This continued attitude will only serve to bring down the entire system.

Subsidizing care is not limited to the illegal immigration problem. The escalation and cost are experienced in other ways through almost all countries. The United States in essence is subsidizing the cost of medication and other pharmaceuticals through drastically inflated prices here in the United States, while other countries pay a fraction of the price paid by us. It is extremely lopsided. Like many things, other countries have taken advantage of the generosity of the United States. This has been perpetuated by the multinational pharmaceutical industry. This practice must stop in order to increase the quality of life in the United States and to allow other countries to pay their fair share. With such an expenditure in pharmaceuticals each year, achieving balance in the open market will greatly decrease one aspect of the American health-care's financial picture.

Trust

Lastly, but much less tangible, American health care, delivery, and financial solvency must have the infusion of much greater trust. This includes the insurance industry, providers, and the consumers/patients. In the present system, the mistrust by all factions and its financial impact of health care is immeasurable. Ronald Reagan once said, "Trust but verify." This is what must happen to promote the

American health-care system and its solvency. No one questions the quality of health care in the United States. It has long been said to be the best in the world. It is the financial aspects which must most importantly be addressed and solved.

CHAPTER 13

Summary

The American health-care system is out of control. This has been universally acknowledged by almost all factions including the insurance industry, providers, consumers, and even politicians. In this acknowledgment very few, if any, faction has stated that the care within the system is subpar. On the contrary, most state that the provision of health care is among the best in the world. The out-of-control spiral comes to the system when looking at the financial aspects of health care. The United States currently spends 3.6 trillion dollars per year on health care, by far the highest expenditure in the world. It is also true the United States is the most generous country in the world. While there are exceptions to every rule, the United States provides health care to all. It has even extended to illegal immigrants to some extent. Blissfully, the people of the United States do not just turn out people with no care when they are unable to pay. It is a credit to the American culture that this is the case; however, without revision, the health-care system will have a certain death.

Various possible steps have been discussed as to what may be needed to fix the cancer that has invaded the system. It is recorded that the health-care system takes 35–42 percent of all health-care dollars to administer health care; yet our neighbor, Canada, does it for half of that percentage. Just the collection of a health-care dollar takes on average 10 percent. Outrageous! Additionally, recent figures place health insurance companies' profit at 8 percent per year.

Imagine, cutting in half the administrative costs and eliminating the insurance companies' yearly profits, the saving through just these two interventions would exceed 1.6 trillion dollars per year. Now couple that savings with all the other interventions discussed, and the health-care expenditure per year would be even more drastically curtailed and well within reasonable societal outlay.

Throughout this book, a number of topics have been explored and the associated symptoms defined. The diagnosis has led to the conclusion that the system is extremely broken and close to life support. It was determined that a number of treatment interventions are necessary to return the system to good health. These interventions are multifaceted. It was also concluded that in large part the delivery of service is good. Like all systems, it can always benefit from improvement and a booster shot. It was determined that it was the financial ramifications of health care that is quickly leading it to insolvency and the need for life support. At best, the system has only used Band-Aids in its treatment, often covering up the real etiology. It was discussed what surgical interventions are deemed necessary to correct its course and return it to a healthy state and to promote ongoing growth. Beyond these interventions, it was clearly evident that all aspects and participants must assist in success. This includes the insurance industry, government, providers, and the American people. Many critics will contend that these interventions are far too simple and the cure is much more complex. These critics will almost always have a horse in this race. Change, or the lack thereof, is mostly political. American society, from the little man all the way up to the highest of high, must ask itself if it has the intestinal fortitude to make the change and return to the American ideal.

ABOUT THE AUTHOR

D r. Richard Cook is a clinical neuropsychologist, a registered vocational rehabilitation consultant, and the Clinical Director and founder of Neuroscience Associates. He is a board-certified forensic examiner and is a Diplomat in Forensic Examination and Forensic Medicine by the American Board of Forensic Examiners and Forensic Medicine. Additionally, he is a Diplomat in Medical Psychology, as well as Forensic Neuropsychology.

He has also been a neuropsychological consultant to the Jimmie Heuga Foundation in Beaver Creek, Colorado, as well as an attending clinical neuropsychologist at Porter Adventist Hospital and North Suburban Medical Center. He also has held consulting privileges at North Valley Rehabilitation Hospital, Colorado Acute Specialty Care Hospital, St. Anthony's Hospital, Kindred Hospital, and Littleton Adventist Hospital.

Dr. Cook completed his doctoral training in clinical psychology in Chicago, Illinois, and subsequently completed his residency training in clinical neuropsychology at Christ Hospital and Medical Center. Dr. Cook has been a neuropsychological consultant and speaker for Eli Lilly and Janssen Pharmaceuticals. He has provided neuropsychological services and consultation in a variety of clinical settings. His breadth of experience includes inpatient, outpatient, and transitional living programs, as well as programs currently under development. Furthermore, he has been an expert witness in both civil and criminal litigation. This has included consultation to numerous insurance companies and defense and plaintiffs' attorneys.

He is a member of numerous professional organizations, including the American Psychological Association, the Council for the National Register of Health Care Providers in Psychology, National

Academy of Neuropsychology, JMA Foundation, National Brain Injury Foundation, National Head Injury Foundation, Colorado Neuropsychological Society, and the American Board of Forensic Examiners. Dr. Cook was chosen to be included in who's who among human service professionals and who's who in America. Finally, he is the author of the *Colorado Cognitive Rehabilitation Series*, copyright 1988–2020, a software program designed for the remediation of cognitive deficits. This program is utilized in rehabilitation programs throughout the country.

CPSIA information can be obtained
at www.ICGtesting.com
Printed in the USA
BVHW070845010821
612698BV00018B/5/J